Exercise Prescription
FOR THE
High-Risk Cardiac Patient

Ray W. Squires, PhD

Mayo Clinic
Division of Cardiovascular Diseases
and Internal Medicine

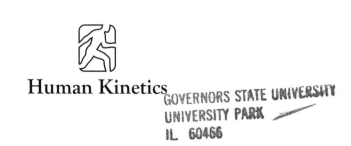

Human Kinetics

Library of Congress Cataloging-in-Publication Data

Squires, Ray White, 1949-
    Exercise prescription for the high-risk cardiac patient / Ray W.
Squires.
      p.   cm.
    Includes bibliographical references and index.
    ISBN 0-87322-980-0
    1. Heart--Diseases--Exercise therapy.   2. Heart--Diseases-
-Exercise therapy--Complications.   3. Heart--Diseases--Patients-
-Rehabilitation.   4. Heart failure--Exercise therapy.   I. Title.
    [DNLM: 1. Myocardial Ischemia--rehabilitation.   2. Exercise
Therapy.   WG 300 S774e 1998]
RC684.E9S67   1998
616.1'2062--DC21
DNLM/DLC
for Library of Congress

97-42640
CIP

ISBN: 0-87322-980-0

Acquisitions Editor: Loarn Robertson; **Developmental Editor:** Kristine Enderle;
Assistant Editor: Laura Hambly; **Copyeditor:** Judy Peterson; **Proofreader:** Erin Cler;
Indexer: Sheila Ary; **Graphic Designer:** Nancy Rasmus; **Graphic Artist:** Denise
Lowry; **Cover Designer:** Jack Davis; **Illustrators:** M.R. Greenberg, Denise Lowry, and
Joe Bellis; **Printer:** Braun-Brumfield

Printed in the United States of America   10   9   8   7   6   5   4   3   2   1

Human Kinetics
Web site: http://www.humankinetics.com/

United States: Human Kinetics, P.O. Box 5076, Champaign, IL 61825-5076
1-800-747-4457
e-mail: humank@hkusa.com

Canada: Human Kinetics, Box 24040, Windsor, ON N8Y 4Y9
1-800-465-7301 (in Canada only)
e-mail: humank@hkcanada.com

Europe: Human Kinetics, P.O. Box IW14, Leeds LS16 6TR, United Kingdom
(44) 1132 781708
e-mail: humank@hkeurope.com

Australia: Human Kinetics, 57A Price Avenue, Lower Mitcham, South Australia 5062
(088) 277 1555
e-mail: humank@hkaustralia.com

New Zealand: Human Kinetics, P.O. Box 105-231, Auckland 1
(09) 523 3462
e-mail: humank@hknewz.com

To my wife, Julia L. Squires, PhD, and to my children:
Lisa, Teresa, Melinda, and Craig.

Contents

Preface

Cardiac rehabilitation, including exercise training, patient and family education and counseling, and risk factor modification has become an accepted component of the care plan for patients with coronary artery disease. Exercise training, an important element of a rehabilitation program, affords important benefits for most cardiac patients, such as these:

- An improvement in exercise capacity and a reduction of symptoms
- Less exercise-related ischemia
- Improvement in classic coronary risk factors
- Improved blood platelet function
- Reduced sympathetic nervous system response to mental and physical stress
- Decreased psychological disturbance and a faster emotional resolution after a cardiac event
- A reduction in the rate of progression of coronary atherosclerosis
- Lower medical care costs
- Improvement in morbidity and mortality for patients with coronary artery disease

Psychological support and control of risk factors such as smoking, dyslipidemia, hypertension, and obesity also significantly benefit the patients participating in a comprehensive cardiac rehabilitation program.

With greater understanding of the benefits of cardiac rehabilitation, the population of patients referred for cardiac rehabilitation services has evolved over the past three decades. At present, a larger number of patients considered at high risk are referred to rehabilitation programs, including patients at risk for complications during exercise testing and training, as well as those at increased risk for recurrent cardiac events including sudden death not temporally related to participation in exercise training. In particular, an increasing number of patients with severe left ventricular dysfunction or large areas of unrevascularizable exercise-induced myocardial ischemia enroll in cardiac rehabilitation programs.

In late 1995, the Agency for Health Care Policy and Research published *Clinical Practice Guideline Number 17: Cardiac Rehabilitation.* This guideline specifically recommends cardiac rehabilitation services, including exercise training, for patients with chronic left ventricular dysfunction resulting from essentially any pathologic condition, that is, coronary artery disease, idiopathic dilated cardiomyopathy, valvular heart disease, hypertension, etc. While some cardiac rehabilitation texts, and a few review articles, provide some information about chronic heart failure and patients with substantial amounts of ischemia, no comprehensive source is currently available. This book proposes to give the reader an in-depth picture of the disease processes, the treatment, and the role of cardiac rehabilitation for patients with chronic left ventricular dysfunction or substantial amounts of myocardial ischemia. Patients with left ventricular dysfunction receive the greater emphasis.

The book is organized into five chapters: defining the high-risk cardiac patient, pathophysiology and treatment options, responses to acute exercise and exercise testing, benefits of exercise training, and suggestions for exercise programming. Specific case studies uniquely illustrate the practical aspects of assessment and formulation of a rehabilitation plan for high-risk cardiac patients.

The intended audience for the book is health care professionals involved in the rehabilitation of cardiac patients, as well as graduate students. It is assumed that the reader has at least a basic understanding of both cardiovascular medicine, and exercise physiology and cardiac rehabilitation. Several excellent texts dealing with cardiac rehabilitation have been recently published (American Association of Cardiovascular and Pulmonary Rehabilitation 1995; American College of Sports Medicine 1995; Fardy and Yanowitz 1995; Pashkow and Dafoe 1993; Pollock and Schmidt 1995; Wenger and Hellerstein 1992); they are recommended for readers who require additional current information regarding the field of cardiac rehabilitation.

References

American Association of Cardiovascular and Pulmonary Rehabilitation. 1995. *Guidelines for Cardiac Rehabilitation Programs*. 2nd ed. Champaign, IL: Human Kinetics.

American College of Sports Medicine. 1995. *Guidelines for Exercise Testing and Exercise Prescription*. 5th ed. Philadelphia: Lea & Febiger.

Fardy PS, Yanowitz FG (Eds.). 1995. *Cardiac Rehabilitation, Adult Fitness, and Exercise Testing*. 3rd ed. Baltimore: Williams & Wilkins.

Pashkow FJ, Dafoe WA (Eds.). 1993. *Clinical Cardiac Rehabilitation: A Cardiologist's Guide*. Baltimore: Williams & Wilkins.

Pollock ML, Schmidt DH (Eds.). 1995. *Heart Disease and Rehabilitation*. 3rd ed. Champaign, IL: Human Kinetics.

U.S. Department of Health and Human Services; Public Health Service; Agency for Health Care Policy and Research; National Heart, Lung, and Blood Institute. 1995. *Clinical Practice Guideline Number 17: Cardiac Rehabilitation* (AHCPR Publication No. 96-0672). Washington, DC: U.S. Government Printing Office.

Wenger NK, Hellerstein HK (Eds.). 1992. *Rehabilitation of the Coronary Patient*. 3rd ed. New York: Churchill-Livingstone.

Acknowledgments

I express appreciation to my secretary, Audrey M. Schroeder, who has provided consistent, professional help and advice throughout this project and has performed a myriad of tasks along the way. Kristine Enderle, my developmental editor at Human Kinetics, efficiently guided the book through the many steps to publication and provided sound, creative, and timely advice. The text and artwork in the book were carefully edited by Laura Hambly of the Human Kinetics staff. I also acknowledge my colleagues at the Mayo Clinic, in particular Gerald T. Gau, M.D., for their contributions to the development of my thinking regarding the evolving discipline of cardiac rehabilitation. Finally, the many patients with severe cardiovascular disease that I have had the pleasure and responsibility with which to work over the years have taught me about their unique problems and have inspired me to write this book.

CHAPTER 1

Defining the High-Risk Cardiac Patient

Patients with cardiovascular disease are a heterogeneous group with various ongoing pathologic processes and differing prognoses. Two important questions for cardiac rehabilitation professionals caring for these patients are, "What is the future risk of a cardiac event or death?" and "What is the risk of an exercise-related medical emergency?"

This chapter discusses many factors that are currently used in risk stratification of patients with cardiovascular disease. It also presents additional novel factors that may become clinically useful in the near future. The potential for exercise-related complications is related to risk stratification factors, although this topic is so important that it merits a separate discussion in the chapter. Patients identified as high risk require a careful evaluation and rehabilitation plan in order to maximize the benefits of rehabilitation while minimizing potential risks.

Clinical Prognostic Factors for Cardiac Patients (Risk Stratification)

The process of risk stratification helps identify patients whose prognosis for future cardiac events and death is high. The following clinical features are particularly important.

Left Ventricular Systolic Function

Left ventricular ejection fraction (LVEF) is the most important prognostic factor in survival for patients with any cardiovascular disease, as has been shown in multiple investigations (Cohn et al. 1993; Emond et al. 1994; Zaret et al. 1995). Figure 1.1 displays the relationship between LVEF and mortality after acute myocardial infarction. For LVEFs below 35%, annual mortality progressively increases to 20% to 30%, or higher.

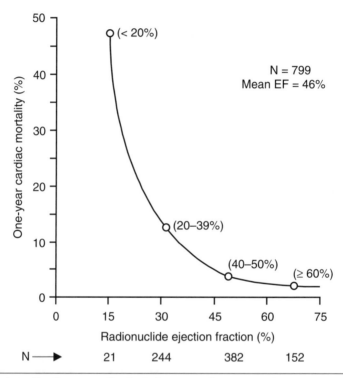

Figure 1.1   Cardiac mortality by left ventricular ejection fraction measured by radionuclide angiography after myocardial infarction.

Survivors of myocardial infarction with LVEFs less than 40% experience a mortality (50% of deaths are sudden) of 20% over 3.5 years (Stevenson and Ridker 1996). LVEF retains its prognostic importance for patients who have received thrombolytic therapy for treatment of acute myocardial infarction. Improvement in LVEF over time has been observed in trials of the treatment of chronic heart failure and results in a more favorable prognosis (see figure 1.2) (Cintron et al. 1993).

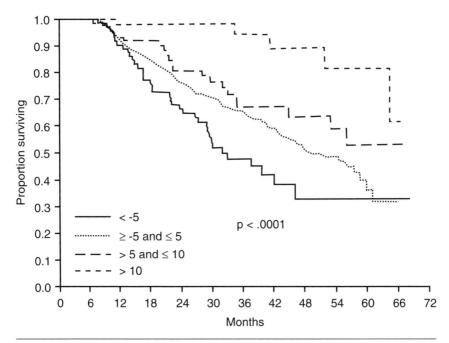

Figure 1.2 Probability of survival over a six-year interval by change in left ventricular ejection fraction.

Reproduced, with permission, from Cintron G, Johnson G, Grancis G, Cobb F, Cohn JN. Prognostic significance of serial changes in left ventricular ejection fraction in patients with congestive heart failure. *Circulation* 87:V1-18. Copyright 1993 American Heart Association.

In general, patients with coronary artery disease have a worse prognosis than those with dilated cardiomyopathy, other factors being equal (Kelly et al. 1990).

Left Ventricular Diastolic Function

Diastolic function, the ability of the left ventricle to fill with blood, is an important determinant of cardiovascular performance, and has prognostic value as well (Belardinelli et al. 1995). In patients with dilated cardiomyopathy, a pattern of abnormal ventricular filling characterized by a higher than normal E wave (peak velocity of early diastolic filling) and a lower than normal A wave (peak velocity of late filling), termed a restrictive pattern by echocardiographers, is associated with a two-year mortality of 60% to 70% (Belardinelli et al. 1995).

Exercise Capacity—$\dot{V}O_2$peak

Exercise test variables, particularly directly measured $\dot{V}O_2$peak (also termed $\dot{V}O_2$max), provide additional well-established prognostic information. Rest LVEF does not predict $\dot{V}O_2$peak. Figure 1.3 shows the relationship

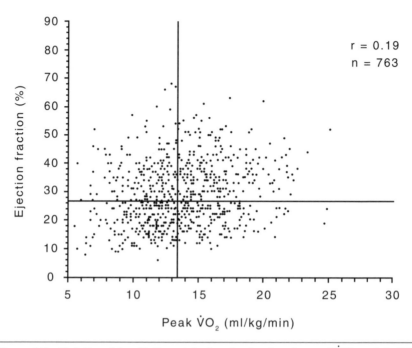

Figure 1.3   Relationship of left ventricular ejection fraction and $\dot{V}O_2$peak in 763 men enrolled in the Department of Veterans Affairs Cooperative Vasodilator—Heart Failure Trial II.

Reproduced, with permission, from Cohn JN, Johnson GR, Shabetai R, Loeb H, Tristani F, Rector T, Smith R, Fletcher R. Ejection fraction, peak exercise oxygen consumption, cardiothoracic ratio, ventricular arrhythmias, and plasma norepinephrine as determinants of prognosis in heart failure. *Circulation* 87:VI-7. Copyright 1993 American Heart Association.

between LVEF and directly measured $\dot{V}O_2$peak for a large cohort of men with varying degrees of chronic heart failure. Note the large variation in $\dot{V}O_2$peak for a given LVEF.

For patients with chronic heart failure and LVEFs below 25%, a $\dot{V}O_2$peak of 14 ml/kg/min or lower carries a poor chance of survival, while a $\dot{V}O_2$peak of > 18 ml/kg/min is associated with an excellent one-year survival (Mancini et al. 1991). Patients with a $\dot{V}O_2$peak of < 10 ml/kg/min have a particularly poor one-year survival (see figure 1.4) (Cohn et al. 1993; Mancini et al. 1991).

The predictive power of $\dot{V}O_2$peak holds true for patients who have suffered a myocardial infarction or who have undergone coronary artery bypass surgery, as shown in figure 1.5 (Vanhees et al. 1994).

Preliminary data suggest improved risk stratification precision using $\dot{V}O_2$peak adjusted for age and gender (Stelkin et al. 1994). This makes intuitive sense, since average $\dot{V}O_2$peak is lower for women than for men and decreases with increasing age, although more data are needed to determine

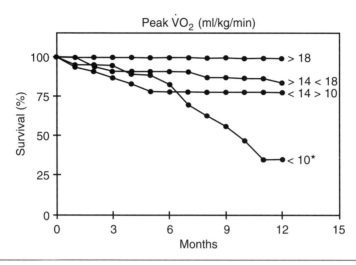

Figure 1.4   Survival curves for chronic heart failure patients with left ventricular ejection fractions of ≤ 25% by peak exercise V̇O₂. ★ p < .05; V̇O₂peak ≤ 10 vs. > 14 ml/kg/min.

Reproduced, with permission, from Mancini DM, Eisen H, Kussmaul W, Mull R, Edmunds LH, Wilson JR. Value of peak exercise oxygen consumption for optimal timing of cardiac transplantation in ambulatory patients with heart failure. *Circulation* 83:783. Copyright 1991 American Heart Association.

new thresholds for risk stratification. A recent investigation using percentage-predicted V̇O₂peak (normalized V̇O₂peak) in 272 ambulatory chronic heart failure patients found only minimal additional prognostic information above and beyond straight V̇O₂peak (Aaronson and Mancini 1995).

The adequacy of the cardiac output increase during exercise may add additional prognostic information beyond the V̇O₂peak measurement (Chomsky et al. 1996). Patients with low left ventricular ejection fractions (mean 22%) who had a normal cardiac output response (measured with hemodynamic lines) to graded exercise experienced a much better one-year survival (95%) than did those with a subnormal cardiac output response (72%, p < .01). However, the worst survival was in patients with a V̇O₂peak of ≤ 10 ml/kg/ min independent of the cardiac output response. Another study including direct cardiac output measurement during graded exercise found very few patients with a normal cardiac output response and did not find additional prognostic information from the measurement (Mancini et al. 1996).

Other Exercise Variables

For patients with chronic heart failure, poor performance (total distance < 300 m) on the six-minute walk test (a field test of exercise capacity described in chapter 3) predicts a high chance of death or hospitalization (Bittner et al. 1993). This finding is particularly meaningful for short-term (six-month) event-free survival (Cahalin et al. 1996).

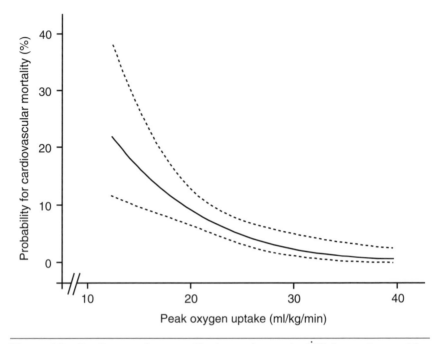

Figure 1.5　Cardiovascular mortality by peak exercise V̇O₂ for patients with a history of myocardial infarction or coronary bypass surgery.

Reprinted from *Journal of the American College of Cardiology*, 23, Vanhees L, Fagard R, Thijs L, Staessen J, Amery A., Prognostic significance of peak exercise capacity in patients with coronary artery disease, 362, Copyright 1994, with permission from the American College of Cardiology.

During graded exercise testing, a drop in systolic blood pressure below preexercise levels is particularly ominous and predicts cardiovascular death or the need for revascularization (Morris et al. 1993).

Myocardial Ischemia

The extent of scintigraphic myocardial ischemia (with exercise thallium perfusion imaging) is also a potent predictor of future cardiovascular events (Mahmarian et al. 1995). Myocardial ischemia assessed with ambulatory ECG monitoring is also predictive of an increased event rate (cardiac death, myocardial infarction, hospital admission for unstable angina, revascularization) in patients after myocardial infarction and with stable angina pectoris (Von Arnim 1996; Gill et al. 1996). Figure 1.6 shows the decrease in event-free survival with increasing transient ischemic episodes during 48-hour ambulatory monitoring. Symptomatic ischemia is associated with more recurrent cardiac events than is painless (silent) ischemia (Narins et al. 1997).

The Duke University treadmill score (derived from treadmill exercise test information), which uses exercise duration, electrocardiographic ST seg-

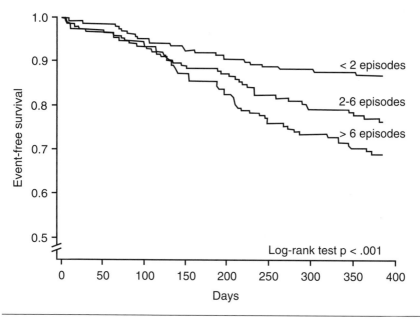

Figure 1.6   Relationship of the number of transient ischemic episodes (48-hour ambulatory ECG monitoring) in 520 patients and event-free survival.

Reprinted from *Journal of the American College of Cardiology*, 28, Von Arnim T. Prognostic significance of transient ischemic episodes: Response to treatment shows improved prognosis: Results of the total ischemic burden bisoprolol study (TIBBS) follow-up, 22, Copyright 1996, with permission from the American College of Cardiology.

ment displacement, and an angina index, is a useful predictor of four-year survival, as shown in table 1.1 (Mark 1994). The Duke treadmill score also predicts nonfatal cardiac events (Pattillo et al. 1996).

Infarct Size

Infarct size, determined approximately one week after acute myocardial infarction using tomographic radionuclide imaging, predicts subsequent mortality and is an important clinical variable. Two-year mortality was 7% in patients whose infarct size was at least 12% of the left ventricle versus 0% for infarct size < 12% in a study from the Mayo Clinic (Miller et al. 1995).

Myocardial Tissue at Risk

The amount of myocardium at risk (viable tissue supplied by a diseased coronary vessel) is also an important predictor of future cardiovascular events (Lee et al. 1994). A larger area of myocardium at risk (especially in the presence of multivessel disease) may represent an unstable substrate for future cardiac events unless it is revascularized. Patients with an open

Table 1.1   Four-Year Survival by Risk Group Based on the Duke Treadmill Score

Risk of death	Inpatients		Outpatients	
	No.	Survival	No.	Survival
Low (≥ +5)	470	0.98	379	0.99
Moderate (-10 to +4)	795	0.92	211	0.95
High (< -10)	129	0.71	23	0.79

The Duke treadmill score is based on three exercise test variables: exercise tolerance in METs, the greatest measured ST segment depression in mm, and an angina pectoris scale (0 = no angina during exercise; 1 = typical angina, 2 = angina requiring test termination). Duke Treadmill Score = (METs - 5[mm ST depression] - 4[treadmill angina score]).

Reprinted from *The American Journal of Cardiology*, 73, Mark DB., An overview of risk assessment in coronary artery disease, 24B, Copyright 1994, with permission from Excerpta Medica Inc.

infarct-related artery (via thrombolytic therapy or spontaneous reperfusion), independent of other clinical characteristics including left ventricular ejection fraction, have a much lower one-year mortality rate than those with an occluded infarct-related artery (Hochman 1996).

Occurrence of Ventricular Fibrillation or Tachycardia (Sudden Cardiac Death)

Survivors of primary (not in the setting of an acute myocardial infarction) ventricular fibrillation or sustained ventricular tachycardia are at high risk for recurrence. Even for patients who have undergone antiarrhythmic drug treatment guided by electrophysiological testing, a recurrence rate of 17% over one year has been reported (Larsen et al. 1994). The greatest event rate occurs during the first month (4%) and the rate decreases over time. Placement of implantable cardioverter-defibrillators improves survival substantially (Osborn 1996).

Additional Prognostic Factors

Several other factors in clinical trials have prognostic importance for patients with chronic heart failure or those who have had a myocardial infarction, although these factors have not been used extensively as yet in clinical practice. Neurohormonal activation as a result of increased sympathetic nervous system tone occurs in the setting of acute myocardial infarction and in chronic heart failure. The plasma concentrations of various peptides resulting from sympathetic activity, such as norepinephrine, renin, aldosterone, atrial naturetic peptide, and arginine vasopressin predict future cardiovascular mortality, the development of severe heart failure, or recurrent myocardial infarction with relative risks of 1.6-2.0 (Rouleau et al. 1994). Figure 1.7 shows the cumulative mortality for chronic heart failure patients with initial plasma norepinephrine concentrations of above or below 900 pg/ml.

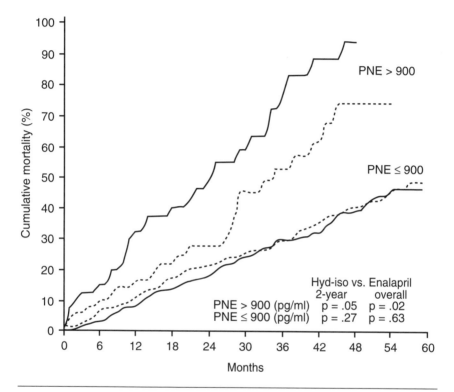

Figure 1.7 Cumulative mortality in patients with chronic heart failure undergoing treatment with vasodilators or angiotensin-converting enzyme inhibitors based on initial plasma norepinephrine (PNE) concentration. ----- = hydralazine + isosorbide dinitrate, ——— = enalapril.

Reproduced, with permission, from Francis GS, Cohn JN, Johnson G, Rector TS, Goldman S, Simon A. Cooperative Studies Group: Plasma norepinephrine, plasma renin activity, and congestive heart failure. *Circulation* 87:I-11. Copyright 1993 American Heart Association.

Plasma sodium concentration, a surrogate measure for renin-angiotensin-aldosterone activation, is strongly associated with prognosis (see figure 1.8). Survival is poor for patients with a plasma sodium of < 138 mmol/L. Concentration in plasma of endothelin, an endothelium-derived vasoconstrictor peptide, is elevated after acute myocardial infarction and is

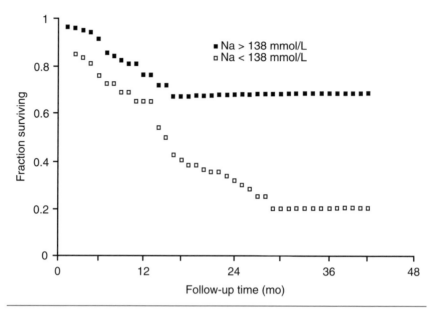

Figure 1.8 Survival of patients with chronic heart failure by plasma sodium concentration.

Reprinted, with permission, from Parameshwar J, Keegan J, Sparrow J, Sutton GC, Poole-Wilson PA. 1992. Predictors of prognosis in severe chronic heart failure. *Am Heart J* 123:421-426.

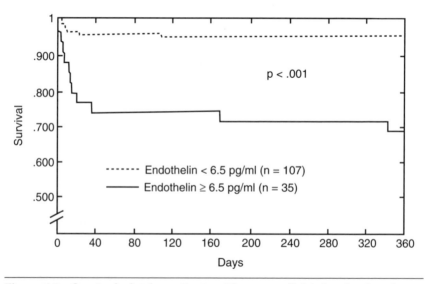

Figure 1.9 Survival plot for patients with myocardial infarction by plasma endothelin concentration above and below the 75th percentile (6.5 pg/ml).

Reproduced, with permission, from Omland T, Lie RT, Aakvaag A, Aarsland T, Dickstein K. Plasma endothelin determination as a prognostic indicator of 1-year mortality after acute myocardial infarction. *Circulation* 89:1575. Copyright 1994 American Heart Association.

strongly predictive of short-term mortality (see figure 1.9). Endothelin concentrations above 6.5 pg/ml are associated with an approximate 30% one-year mortality.

A shift in the leukocyte differential toward a decrease in the percentage of lymphocytes predicts increased one- and five-year survival in chronic heart failure patients (Ommen et al. 1997). This most likely reflects an increased production of cortisol due to the physiologic stress of illness.

Heart rate variability, which is a function of the interplay between the parasympathetic (increases heart rate variability) and sympathetic (decreases heart rate variability) divisions of the autonomic nervous system, is reduced after myocardial infarction and is associated with an increase in subsequent cardiac death and all-cause mortality (Mattioni 1992). Decreased fibrinolytic activity is associated with a poor prognosis after myocardial infarction. In particular, elevated plasma plasminogen activator inhibitor-1 concentrations (> 20 U/ml) reduce fibrinolytic potential and predict reinfarction and cardiac death (Malmberg et al. 1994).

Psychosocial Factors

Various psychological factors predict future cardiac events. Depression present after myocardial infarction carries an ominous 20% mortality over 18 months compared with 6% for similar patients without depression (Frasure-Smith et al. 1995). Psychological distress of a general nature is associated with higher rates of rehospitalization, recurrent myocardial infarction, cardiac arrest with resuscitation, and cardiac death (Allison et al. 1995). Social isolation (living alone) after myocardial infarction is also associated with a doubling of recurrent cardiac events during the first six months of recovery (Case et al. 1992).

Additional psychosocial factors such as a high work load, multiple chronic nonspecific complaints, and failure to identify disease-promoting factors within lifestyle or surroundings have been suggested to predict a poor prognosis after myocardial infarction (Hoffman et al. 1995).

Gender Differences

A commonly held belief is that women have a higher late mortality than men after myocardial infarction. In fact, survival after myocardial infarction is similar for women and men after adjusting for other factors such as left ventricular function, ventricular arrhythmias, and sympathetic nervous system activation (Gottlieb et al. 1994).

Women with nonischemic symptomatic left ventricular dysfunction generally experience a better survival than do men (Adams et al. 1996). Women and men have a similar survival if the cause of the chronic heart failure is coronary artery disease. In addition, patients of either gender whose symptoms are relatively stable have a more favorable prognosis than do patients with worsening symptoms (Rickenbacher et al. 1996).

Of all the clinical factors, the following have been identified as established powerful predictors of a poor prognosis for cardiac patients:

- Left ventricular systolic dysfunction; left ventricular ejection fraction equal to or less than 35%, congestive heart failure symptoms
- Large myocardial infarction (involving > 35% of the left ventricle), large anterior wall myocardial infarction
- Poor exercise capacity; peak oxygen uptake less than 14 ml/kg/min (4 METs)
- Evidence of extensive, severe ischemia during exercise or pharmacological stress testing
- Primary sudden cardiac death (not associated with acute myocardial infarction); previous ventricular fibrillation or sustained ventricular tachycardia
- Extensive, severe obstructive coronary atherosclerosis (left main, proximal left anterior descending, severe three-vessel disease) that is not revascularized

Physical Activity and Exercise for Cardiac Patients

Regular exercise training has been conclusively demonstrated to protect individuals from myocardial infarction and cardiac death (Powell et al. 1987). However, physical activity for cardiac patients is acutely associated with a transient increase in the risk of developing myocardial ischemia, myocardial infarction, and sudden cardiac death (Meissner et al. 1991). By increasing myocardial oxygen requirement, exercise may result in ischemia in patients with fixed atherosclerotic lesions or in patients with vasospasm.

Myocardial ischemia, whether progressing to myocyte necrosis or not, is an important causative factor for cardiac arrest. However, lethal ventricular arrhythmias do occur independent of acute ischemia, probably related to myocardial scarring from previous infarction.

Mittleman et al. (1993) interviewed 1,228 patients who suffered and survived an acute myocardial infarction. In approximately 5% of patients, heavy physical exertion apparently triggered the infarction, presumably by increased hemodynamic stress causing rupture of a vulnerable atherosclerotic plaque leading to formation of an occlusive thrombus. Because myocardial infarction and sudden cardiac death are more common in the early morning hours than in the afternoon (see figure 1.10), investigators have determined that physical exertion plays an important causative role.

Parker et al. (1994) studied 20 patients with coronary artery disease with ambulatory ECG monitoring. The investigators altered the normal morning

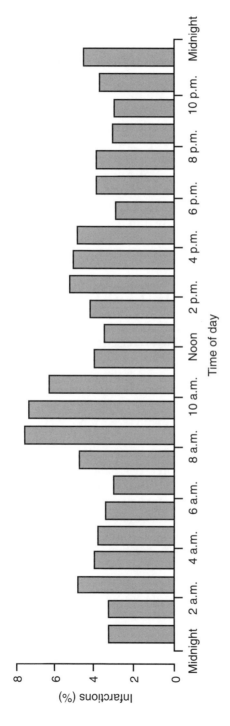

Figure 1.10 Time distribution of the onset of acute myocardial infarction in 1,194 patients. Adapted, with permission, from Willich SN, Lewis M, Lowell H, Arntz HR, Schubert F, Schroder R. Physical exertion as a trigger of acute myocardial infarction. *N Eng J Med* 329:1684-1690. Copyright 1993 Massachusetts Medical Society. All rights reserved.

pattern of physical activity by keeping the patients sedentary until almost noon. Compared with normal morning activity patterns, heart rate remained lower and episodes of ischemia were delayed until physical activity began in the afternoon. Thus, exercise may be considered an acute risk factor for a cardiac event (Muller et al. 1994).

Is early morning, rather than afternoon or evening, exercise training more dangerous for cardiac patients? Murray et al. (1993) surveyed cardiac rehabilitation exercise programs with either early morning or afternoon exercise classes. Over approximately ten years of observation, 168,111 and 84,491 patient-hours of exercise were performed, respectively, by the morning and afternoon groups. Event rates (ventricular fibrillation, cardiac syncope) were similar for the morning (3.0 events per 100,000 patient-hours of exercise) and afternoon programs (2.4 events per 100,000 patient-hours of exercise) and were not significantly different. Early morning regular exercise training is not associated with an increased risk of myocardial infarction or sudden cardiac death.

Exercise-Related Complications

Van Camp and Peterson (1986) surveyed 167 cardiac rehabilitation programs in the early 1980s regarding exercise-related cardiac complications. Included in their report was a cohort of 51,303 patients who performed 2,351,916 hours of supervised exercise training. Cardiac arrest was documented in 21 cases (1 event per 111,996 patient-hours of exercise) and myocardial infarction in 8 cases (1 infarction per 293,990 patient-hours of exercise). Surprisingly, only three deaths were reported (1 death per 783,972 patient-hours of exercise) indicative of an excellent rate of successful resuscitation. The patients included in this study were not further risk stratified, and the rate of complication for high-risk patients was not reported.

However, Van Camp and Peterson (1989) subsequently analyzed the clinical characteristics of 20 of the 29 patients with a serious complication from the original cohort. All had coronary artery disease. A substantial number of high-risk characteristics were prevalent: prior cardiac arrest (n = 4), prior ventricular tachycardia (n = 6), history of congestive heart failure (n = 3), left ventricular ejection fraction < 40% (n = 3), signs of exercise-induced ischemia (n = 5), and left main or severe three-vessel disease (not revascularized, n = 6). From these data, it appears that serious complications during exercise training are much more prevalent in high-risk patients.

Risk Stratification for Exercise-Related Complications

The American Heart Association, with the endorsement of the American College of Sports Medicine, has recommended that the following clinical factors be used to identify patients at higher risk (class D) for a serious exercise-related complication such as acute myocardial infarction or sudden cardiac death (Fletcher et al. 1995):

- Severe coronary artery disease
  1. History of two or more myocardial infarctions
  2. New York Heart Association class 3 or higher heart failure symptoms
  3. Exercise capacity less than 6 METs
  4. Ischemic horizontal or downsloping ST segment depression of at least 4.0 mm, or angina during exercise
  5. Fall in systolic blood pressure during exercise testing
  6. Life-threatening medical problem (physician determined)
  7. Previous episode of primary cardiac arrest
  8. Ventricular tachycardia occurring at an exercise intensity of less than 6 METs
- Cardiomyopathy
- Valvular heart disease (severe)
- Exercise test abnormalities not directly related to ischemia
- Previous episode of ventricular fibrillation or cardiac arrest not related to the presence of an acute cardiac event or cardiac procedure
- Complex ventricular arrhythmias uncontrolled at mild to moderate intensities of exercise
- Three-vessel or left main disease
- LVEFs less than 30%

As can be easily appreciated, considerable overlap exists between the factors listed above for exercise-related risk and the ones discussed previously regarding general prognosis.

Serious exercise-related complications include symptomatic sustained ventricular tachycardia, ventricular fibrillation, acute myocardial infarction, hemodynamically compromising bradyarrhythmias, atrioventricular dissociation, high-grade atrioventricular block, pulmonary edema, and any other condition resulting in cardiac syncope. The literature includes surprisingly few published reports regarding the rate of serious complications during cardiac rehabilitation program-based exercise training. No such data are available specifically for high-risk patients, presumably due to the relatively small numbers of these patients involved in supervised exercise training.

Conclusion: The High-Risk Patient

Based upon the forgoing discussion of factors implicated in predicting either future cardiac events related or nonrelated to acute exercise, the following characteristics (one or more) are suggested for the definition of a high-risk patient:

- Left ventricular ejection fraction less than or equal to 35%, or congestive heart failure due primarily to diastolic dysfunction
- Extremely poor exercise capacity; directly measured $\dot{V}O_2$peak less than 14 ml/kg/min
- Evidence of extensive, severe myocardial ischemia during exercise or pharmacological stress testing
- Survivor of primary sudden cardiac death without treatment with an implantable cardioverter-defibrillator
- Severe unrevascularizable coronary artery disease (left main, severe proximal three-vessel disease)

The remainder of the book deals with rehabilitation issues for these interesting, albeit complicated patients. Case study material also illustrates potential rehabilitation of patients with rare conditions (amyloid heart disease) or disease that is usually considered an absolute contraindication to exercise training (severe aortic stenosis, obstructive hypertrophic cardiomyopathy).

References

Aaronson KD, Mancini DM. 1995. Is percentage of predicted maximal exercise oxygen consumption a better predictor of survival than peak exercise oxygen consumption for patients with severe heart failure? *J Heart Lung Transplant* 14:981-989.

Adams KF, Dunlap SH, Sueta CA, Clarke SW, Patterson JH, Blauwet MB, Jensen LR, Tomasko L, Koch G. 1996. Relation between gender, etiology and survival in patients with symptomatic heart failure. *J Am Coll Cardiol* 28:1781-1788.

Allison TG, Williams DE, Miller TD, Patten CA, Bailey KR, Squires RW, Gau GT. 1995. Medical and economic costs of psychological distress in patients with coronary artery disease. 1995. *Mayo Clin Proc* 70:734-742.

Belardinelli R, Georgiou D, Cianci G, Berman N, Ginzton L, Purcaro A. 1995. Exercise training improves left ventricular diastolic filling in patients with dilated cardiomyopathy: Clinical and prognostic implications. *Circulation* 91:2775-2784.

Bittner V, Weiner DH, Yusuf S, Rogers WJ, McIntyre KM, Bangdiwala SI, Kronenberg MW, Kostis JB, Kohn RM, Guillotte M, Greenberg B, Woods PA, Bourassa MG. 1993. Prediction of mortality and morbidity with a six-minute walk test in patients with left ventricular dysfunction. *JAMA* 270:1702-1707.

Cahalin LP, Mathier MA, Semigran MJ, Dec GW, DiSalvo TG. 1996. The six-minute walk test predicts peak oxygen uptake and survival in patients with advanced heart failure. *Chest* 110:325-332.

Case RB, Moss AJ, Case N, McDermott M, Eberly S. 1992. Living alone after myocardial infarction: Impact on prognosis. *JAMA* 267:515-519.

Chomsky DB, Lang CC, Rayos GH, Shyr Y, Yeoh TK, Pierson RN, Davis SF, Wilson JR. 1996. Hemodynamic exercise testing: A valuable tool in the selection of cardiac transplantation candidates. *Circulation* 94:3176-3183.

Cintron G, Johnson G, Francis G, Cobb F, Cohn JN. 1993. Prognostic significance of serial changes in left ventricular ejection fraction in patients with congestive heart failure. *Circulation* 87(Suppl VI):17-23.

Cohn JN, Johnson GR, Shabetai R, Loeb H, Tristani F, Rector T, Smith R, Fletcher R. 1993. Ejection fraction, peak exercise oxygen consumption, cardiothoracic ratio, ventricular arrhythmias, and plasma norepinephrine as determinants of prognosis in heart failure. *Circulation* 87(Suppl VI):5-16.

Emond M, Mock MB, Davis KB, Fisher LD, Holmes DR, Chaitman BR, Kaiser GC, Alderman E, Killip T. 1994. Long-term survival of medically treated patients in the coronary artery surgery study (CASS) registry. *Circulation* 90:2645-2657.

Fletcher GF, Balady G, Froelicher VF, Hartley LH, Haskell WL, Pollock ML. 1995. Exercise standards: A statement for health care professionals from the American Heart Association. *Circulation* 91:580-615.

Frasure-Smith N, Lesperance F, Talajk M. 1995. Depression and 18-month prognosis after myocardial infarction. *Circulation* 91:999-1005.

Gill JB, Cairns JA, Roberts RS, Costantini L, Sealey BJ, Fallen EF, Tomlinson CW, Gent M. 1996. Prognostic importance of myocardial ischemia detected by ambulatory monitoring early after acute myocardial infarction. *N Eng J Med* 334:65-70.

Gottlieb S, Moss AJ, McDermott M, Eberly S. 1994. Comparison of posthospital survival after acute myocardial infarction in women and men. *Am J Cardiol* 74:727-730.

Hochman JS. 1996. Has the time come to seek and open all occluded infarct-related arteries after myocardial infarction? *J Am Coll Cardiol* 28:846-848.

Hoffman A, Pfiffner D, Hornung R, Niederhauser H. 1995. Psychosocial factors predict medical outcome following a first myocardial infarction. *Coronary Artery Disease* 6:147-152.

Kelly TS, Cremo R, Neilsen C, Shabetai R. 1990. Prediction of outcome in late-stage cardiomyopathy. *Am Heart J* 119:1111-1121.

Larsen GC, Stupey MR, Walance CG, Griffith KK, Cutler JE, Kron J, McAnulty JH. 1994. Recurrent cardiac events in survivors of ventricular fibrillation or tachycardia: Implications for driving restrictions. *JAMA* 271:1335-1339.

Lee KS, Marwick TH, Cook SA, Go RT, Fix JS, James KB, Sapp SK, MacIntyre WJ, Thomas JD. 1994. Prognosis of patients with left ventricular dysfunction, with and without viable myocardium after myocardial infarction: Relative efficacy of medical therapy and revascularization. *Circulation* 90:2687-2694.

Mahmarian JJ, Mahmarian AC, Marks GF, Pratt CM, Verani MS. 1995. Role of adenosine thallium-201 tomography for defining long-term risk in patients after acute myocardial infarction. *J Am Coll Cardiol* 25:1333-1340.

Malmberg K, Barenholm P, Hamsten A. 1994. Clinical and biochemical factors associated with prognosis after myocardial infarction at a young age. *J Am Coll Cardiol* 24:592-599.

Mancini DM, Eisen H, Kussmaul W, Mull R, Edmunds LH, Wilson JR. 1991. Value of peak exercise oxygen consumption for optimal timing of cardiac transplantation in ambulatory patients with heart failure. *Circulation* 83:778-786.

Mancini DM, Katz S, Donchez L, Aaronson K. 1996. Coupling of hemodynamic measurements with oxygen consumption during exercise does not improve risk stratification in patients with heart failure. *Circulation* 94:2492-2496.

Mark DB. 1994. An overview of risk assessment in coronary artery disease. *Am J Cardiol* 73:19B-25B.

Mattioni TA. 1992. Long-term prognosis after myocardial infarction: Who is at risk for sudden death? *Postgrad Med* 92:107-114.

Meissner MD, Akhtar M, Lehman MH. 1991. Nonischemic sudden tachyarrhythmic death in atherosclerotic heart disease. *Circulation* 84:905-912.

Miller TD, Christian TF, Hopfenspirger MR, Hodge DO, Gersh BJ, Gibbons RJ. 1995. Infarct size after acute myocardial infarction measured by quantitative tomographic ^{99m}Tc sestamibi imaging predicts subsequent mortality. *Circulation* 92:334-341.

Mittleman MA, Maclure M, Tofler GH, Sherwood JB, Goldberg RJ, Muller JE. 1993. Triggering of acute myocardial infarction by heavy physical exertion: Protection against triggering by regular exertion. *N Eng J Med* 329:1677-1683.

Morris CK, Morrow K, Froelicher VF, Hideg A, Hunter D, Kawaguchi T, Ribisl PM, Ueshima K, Wallis J. 1993. Prediction of cardiovascular death by means of clinical and exercise test variables in patients selected for cardiac catheterization. *Am Heart J* 125:1717-1726.

Muller JE, Abela GS, Nesto RW, Tofler GH. 1994. Triggers, acute risk factors and vulnerable plaques: The lexicon of a new frontier. *J Am Coll Cardiol* 23:809-813.

Murray PM, Herrington DM, Pettus CW, Miller HS, Cantwell JD, Little WC. 1993. Should patients with heart disease exercise in the morning or afternoon? *Arch Intern Med* 153:833-836.

Narins CR, Zareba W, Moss AJ, Goldstein RE, Hall WJ. 1997. Clinical implications of silent versus symptomatic exercise-induced myocardial ischemia in patients with stable coronary disease. *J Am Coll Cardiol* 29:756-763.

Ommen SR, Hodge DO, Rodeheffer RJ, McGregor CGA, Thomson SP, Gibbons RJ. 1997. The relative lymphocyte concentration: A new prognostic marker in end-stage heart failure. *J Am Coll Cardiol* 29(Suppl A):102A.

Osborn MJ. 1996. Sudden cardiac death. A. Mechanisms, incidence and prevention of sudden cardiac death. In *Mayo Clinic Practice of Cardiology*. 3rd ed. Giuliani ER, Gersh BJ, McGoon MD, Hayes DL, Schaff HV (eds). St. Louis: Mosby, pp. 862-894.

Parker JD, Testa MA, Jimenez AH, Tofler GH, Muler JE, Parker JO, Stone PH. 1994. Morning increase in ambulatory ischemia in patients with stable coronary artery disease: Importance of physical activity and increased cardiac demand. *Circulation* 89:604-614.

Pattillo RW, Fuchs S, Johnson J, Cave V, Heo J, DePace NL, Iskandrain AS. 1996. Predictors of prognosis by quantitative assessment of coronary angiography, single photon emission computed tomography thallium imaging, and treadmill exercise testing. *Am Heart J* 131:582-590.

Powell KE, Thompson PD, Caspersen CJ, Kendrick JS. 1987. Physical activity and the incidence of coronary heart disease. *Ann Rev Public Health* 8:253-287.

Rickenbacher PR, Trindade PT, Haywood GA, Vagelos RH, Schroeder JS, Willson K, Prikazsky L, Fowler MB. 1996. Transplant candidates with severe left ventricular dysfunction managed with medical treatment: Characteristics and survival. *J Am Coll Cardiol* 27:1192-1197.

Rouleau JL, Packer M, Moye L, deChamplain J, Bichet D, Klein M, Rouleau JR, Sussex B, Arnold JM, Sestier F, Parker JO, McEwan P, Bernstein V, Cuddy TE, Lamas G, Gottlieb SS, McCans J, Nadeau C, Delage F, Wun CC, Pfeffer MA. 1994. Prognostic value of neurohormonal activation in patients with an acute myocardial infarction: Effect of Captopril. *J Am Coll Cardiol* 24:583-591.

Stelkin AM, Younis LT, Jennison SH, Wolford T, Miller LW, Miller DD, Chaitman BR. 1994. Improved risk stratification of ambulatory congestive heart failure patients using age and gender adjusted percent predicted peak exercise oxygen uptake. *J Am Coll Cardiol* 23(Abstract):448.

Stevenson WG, Ridker PM. 1996. Should survivors of myocardial infarction with low ejection fraction be routinely referred to arrhythmia specialists? *JAMA* 276:481-485.

Van Camp SP, Peterson RA. 1986. Cardiovascular complications of outpatient cardiac rehabilitation programs. *JAMA* 256:1160-1163.

Van Camp SP, Peterson RA. 1989. Identification of the high-risk cardiac rehabilitation patient. *J Cardiopulm Rehabil* 9:103-109.

Vanhees L, Fagard R, Thijs L, Staessen J, Amery A. 1994. Prognostic significance of peak exercise capacity in patients with coronary artery disease. *J Am Coll Cardiol* 23:358-363.

Von Arnim T. 1996. Prognostic significance of transient ischemic episodes: Response to treatment shows improved prognosis: Results of the total ischemic burden bisoprolol study (TIBBS) follow-up. *J Am Coll Cardiol* 28:20-24.

Zaret BL, Wackers FJT, Terrin ML, Forman SA, Williams DO, Knatterud GL, Braunwald E. 1995. Value of radionuclide rest and exercise left ventricular ejection fraction in assessing survival of patients after thrombolytic therapy for acute myocardial infarction: Results of thrombolysis in myocardial infarction (TIMI) phase II study. *J Am Coll Cardiol* 26:73-79.

CHAPTER 2

Pathophysiology and Treatment of Myocardial Ischemia and Chronic Heart Failure
(Left Ventricular Dysfunction)

Most high-risk patients referred to cardiac rehabilitation programs will have myocardial ischemia resulting from coronary artery disease (CAD) or chronic heart failure (left ventricular dysfunction). This chapter highlights the underlying pathology of these disorders and provides insight into the comprehensive approach to their treatment. An in-depth discussion of the benefits of exercise training for patients with myocardial ischemia or chronic heart failure appears in chapter 4.

Coronary Atherosclerosis

Atherosclerosis of the coronary arteries (coronary artery disease) is a progressive, multifactorial disease with many established risk factors, such as cigarette smoking, an adverse blood lipid profile (elevated non-HDL cholesterol, low HDL cholesterol, elevated triglycerides, elevated Lp(a), etc.), hypertension, sedentary lifestyle, genetic predisposition, diabetes mellitus, psychological disturbance, male gender, and increasing age (Squires and Williams 1993).

Coronary artery disease (CAD) begins with injury to the endothelial layer of the artery with a subsequent inflammatory response leading to infiltration of monocytes into the intimal layer of the vessel, release of growth factors from platelets, incorporation of cholesterol and other substances from the blood, migration of smooth muscle cells from the vessel media, plaque formation, and thrombi formation on the plaque at sites of fissuring or rupture, leading to progressive obstruction of blood flow through the affected artery (Ross 1988). Figure 2.1 provides an overview of the atherosclerotic process.

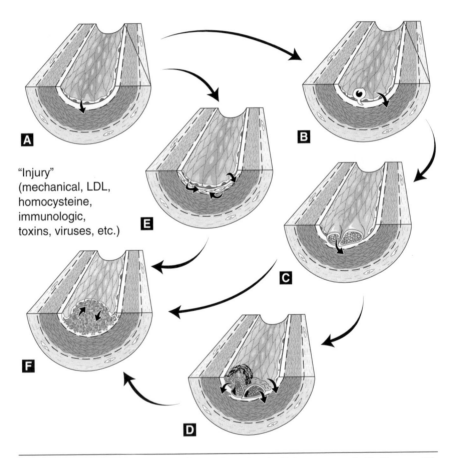

"Injury"
(mechanical, LDL,
homocysteine,
immunologic,
toxins, viruses, etc.)

Figure 2.1 The process of atherosclerosis. A. Injury to endothelium with release of growth factors (small arrow). B. Monocytes attach to endothelium. C. Monocytes migrate to the intima, take up cholesterol, form fatty streaks. D. Platelets adhere to endothelium and release growth factors. F. The result is a fibromuscular plaque. An alternative pathway is shown with arrows from A to E to F, with growth factor-mediated migration of smooth cells from media to the intima (E).

Coronary atherosclerosis affects vessels in a diffuse manner with occasional, discrete localized areas of more pronounced narrowing that may impede blood flow. A substantial reduction in vessel internal diameter may occur before a decrease in blood flow at rest can be measured distal to the plaque. When luminal cross-sectional area is reduced by 75% or more, blood flow at rest will be impaired. Beyond this critical degree of stenosis, further seemingly small decreases in cross-sectional area will result in marked further reductions in flow. The reduction in cross-sectional area may be caused by atherosclerotic plaque, alone or in concert with platelet aggregation, leading to thrombus formation and vasospasm due to contraction of vascular smooth muscle (Lie 1991).

Normal myocardial contraction and relaxation is dependent upon adequate amounts of high-energy phosphate (ATP) supplies in cardiac muscle. The heart produces ATP with aerobic metabolism under normal conditions, and is not adapted to produce many ATP molecules anaerobically. During exercise, the oxygen requirement of the myocardium may increase 200% to 300% above resting conditions (Garratt and Morgan 1991).

Because the myocardium extracts nearly all of the available oxygen from the arterial blood that flows through its capillary beds, coronary blood flow must be up- or down-regulated precisely to meet the needs of the myocardium for oxygen (Guyton 1986). With an increase in myocardial work, coronary blood flow must be augmented to deliver the required amount of oxygen. Under normal conditions the autonomic nervous system and local substances produced within the myocardium or coronary vessels regulate coronary flow by altering the caliber of resistance vessels in accordance with myocardial need for oxygen.

Myocardial Ischemia

Myocardial ischemia is defined as inadequate blood flow (inadequate myocardial perfusion) to supply the necessary amount of oxygen for the heart (Braunwald and Sobel 1988). Myocardial ischemia causes relative oxygen deprivation accompanied by inadequate removal of various metabolites. The following physiological abnormalities result from ischemia:

- Hypoxia (insufficient oxygen for the needs of aerobic production of ATP)
- Accumulation of toxic metabolites
- Development of acidosis

Hypoxia slows aerobic metabolism and the intracellular stores of ATP may become depleted. This results in a shift from aerobic to anaerobic production of ATP accompanied by a dramatic increase in lactic acid formation causing acidosis. Under ischemic conditions, the heart releases lactate into the venous blood.

Myocardial ischemia may be diagnosed by an electrocardiogram either during symptoms, with a 24-hour ambulatory recording, or during graded exercise testing. Additional techniques used to detect ischemia include radionuclide perfusion or echocardiography during exercise, and positron emission tomography.

Ischemic Cascade

Myocardial ischemia may result in progressive abnormalities in cardiac function referred to as the ischemic cascade (Hurst 1992). The first abnormality is stiffening of the left ventricle, which reduces the ability of the chamber to fill with blood during diastole (diastolic dysfunction).

As cardiac function degenerates, systolic function, namely ventricular emptying and stroke volume, becomes impaired. This is the second cardiac abnormality resulting from myocardial ischemia. Localized areas of the myocardium may develop asynergistic contraction patterns such as hypokinesis (reduced systolic contraction), akinesis (absent contraction), or dyskinesis (paradoxical aneurysmic bulging of a segment of myocardium during contraction).

During normal cardiac function, the ventricular myocytes shorten during systole and cause the ventricular walls to thicken and move forward as contraction proceeds. During ischemia, altered systolic function may develop and cause segmental wall-motion contraction abnormalities and a reduction in left ventricular ejection fraction and stroke volume.

The third abnormality is manifested by electrocardiographic changes associated with altered repolarization (ST segment elevation or depression, T wave inversion) as a result of nonuniform repolarization through the ischemic and surrounding normal tissue. Ischemia may initiate serious ventricular arrhythmia.

Finally, the patient may develop symptoms of angina pectoris. Some patients with severe ischemia do not develop symptoms (silent ischemia).

Angina Pectoris

The locations and sensations of angina pectoris are diverse (Shub 1991). Anginal pain is usually located in the substernal region, jaw, neck, or left arm, although a sensation may occur in the epigastrium and interscapular regions. The sensation is often described as a pressure, heaviness, fullness, squeezing, burning, aching, or choking. The pain may vary in intensity and may radiate.

Impairment of ventricular contraction and relaxation due to ischemia may result in elevated left ventricular filling pressures (increased end-diastolic pressure). A back pressure in the pulmonary circulation leading to pulmonary congestion and dyspnea (anginal equivalent) may result.

Angina is usually provoked by exertion, emotions, cold or heat exposure, meals, and sexual intercourse, and is relieved by rest or nitroglycerin.

Unstable angina is defined as a new onset of exertional angina, increasing frequency or intensity or duration of previously stable angina, or angina that occurs at rest (Shub 1991). Unstable angina is thought to be the result of plaque rupture with the subsequent development of transient platelet thrombi (thrombi that form and then dissolve), or periodic vasospasm mediated by local vasoconstrictors such as endothelin (Chesebro et al. 1991).

Rupture of a plaque with subsequent occlusive thrombus formation may result in severe, prolonged ischemia with irreversible myocyte damage (infarction). If ischemia is merely transient (less than 60 minutes), postischemic ventricular dysfunction may be present for hours to days and is termed stunned myocardium. With more lengthy periods of ischemia, myocytes may remain viable but do not contract normally, a situation called hibernating myocardium (Ferrari 1995). This phenomenon appears to be a protective mechanism whereby myocytes reduce their oxygen demand when the oxygen supply is inadequate for normal function. After reperfusion, as with revascularization, contractile function may return to normal immediately or it may gradually return over a period of time up to one year in length (Rahimtoola 1995).

Treatment for Myocardial Ischemia

Myocardial ischemia may be treated with medications, revascularization procedures, risk factor modification, and exercise training. All patients with coronary artery disease should be considered candidates for aggressive risk factor reduction and regular physical activity. The choice of medical and surgical treatment is not always clear-cut.

Medical Treatment

Medical treatment of myocardial ischemia is designed to increase myocardial blood flow, reduce myocardial oxygen requirement, decrease arrhythmia, improve platelet and endothelial function, and impair thrombus formation. In addition, some drugs and vitamins may directly decrease the progression of coronary atherosclerosis.

Nitroglycerin

Nitroglycerin is an effective treatment for symptoms and objective markers of myocardial ischemia such as electrocardiographic and imaging (nuclear scans, echocardiography) abnormalities. Mechanisms of action for nitroglycerin include the following:

- Coronary vasodilation, which potentially improves myocardial oxygen supply
- Systemic vasodilation, which reduces afterload and left ventricular end-diastolic pressure

- An antiplatelet effect that inhibits platelet aggregation and increases induced disaggregation of developed platelet thrombi (Bertolet and Pepine 1995).

Beta Adrenergic Blockers

Beta adrenergic blockers reduce myocardial oxygen demand by lowering heart rate and blood pressure at rest and during exercise. In addition, they are effective antiarrhythmics and have antiplatelet action. After myocardial infarction, beta blockers improve survival and their use postinfarction is a standard of care.

Calcium Channel Antagonists

Calcium channel antagonists reduce blood pressure, prevent vasospasm, and for some of the drugs, reduce heart rate. They are somewhat less effective in reducing ischemia than are beta blockers. They may also inhibit platelet thrombus formation.

Antiplatelet Drugs

Aspirin is a platelet inhibitor that has been demonstrated to reduce ischemic events. Ticlopidine, a thromboxane A2 inhibitor, also reduces ischemic episodes.

Combination Therapy

Combination therapy with nitrates, beta blockers, calcium channel antagonists, and aspirin is an effective treatment strategy for many patients with myocardial ischemia, especially those patients who are not candidates for complete revascularization (McGoon and Shub 1996).

Angiotensin-Converting Enzyme Inhibitors

Angiotensin-converting enzyme inhibitors improve endothelial dysfunction even in patients with CAD who are normotensive and do not have evidence of heart failure (Mancini et al. 1996). The improvement in endothelial dysfunction may be additive to the similar effect described for the drugs for lipid lowering (Pitt 1997). Thus, this class of medications may have an expanding role in the treatment of myocardial ischemia in the future.

Estrogen

Estrogen replacement for postmenopausal women with CAD should be carefully considered (Stevenson et al. 1994; Gerhard and Ganz 1995; Guetta and Cannon 1996). Estrogen increases high-density lipoprotein cholesterol and lowers low-density lipoprotein cholesterol, which favorably affects atherosclerosis and ischemia, as will be discussed later in this chapter. Estrogen also corrects endothelial dysfunction seen in the setting of atherosclerosis, reduces blood pressure, possesses antioxidant effects, lowers plasma fibrinogen levels and elevates tissue plasminogen activator concentrations, decreases myocardial ischemia during exercise, limits the development of central obesity, and improves insulin resistance. The concurrent use of progestins in women with an intact uterus does not appear to markedly reduce the potential cardioprotective effects of estrogen replacement (Grodstein et al. 1996). However, randomized clinical trials (currently in progress) are necessary before the benefits and limitations of estrogen replacement are fully understood (Rossouw 1996).

Vitamin Supplementation

Vitamin supplementation appears to be beneficial for patients with coronary artery disease. The Cambridge heart antioxidant study (CHAOS) randomized 2,002 coronary patients to vitamin E supplementation (400 or 800 IU qd) or placebo (Stephens et al. 1996). Over an average of 510 days of follow-up, the treatment group demonstrated a significantly lower incidence of nonfatal myocardial infarction. Vitamin C may reverse endothelial dysfunction seen in patients with atherosclerosis (Levine et al. 1996), although the effect on daily ischemia or cardiovascular events is not known.

Revascularization Procedures

Direct revascularization of ischemic myocardium is extremely effective in reducing or eliminating ischemia and its related symptoms.

Catheter-Based Revascularization

Catheter-based revascularization with balloon angioplasty, stents, directional atherectomy, laser angioplasty, and rotablator is a rapidly evolving field. The main limitation of these forms of treatment is restenosis of the coronary segment that underwent manipulation (Garratt et al. 1996).

Bypass Surgery

Coronary artery bypass surgery using saphenous veins and internal thoracic or radial arteries as conduits is a highly effective treatment for selected patients (McGoon et al. 1996). The primary limitation of surgical intervention is a three-month recuperation. However, new techniques using a mini-thoracotomy or endoscopic entry into the thorax allow placement of a left internal thoracic artery to left anterior descending anastamosis without a sternotomy. The circumflex or right coronary artery could then conceivably be treated with angioplasty in selected cases.

Transmyocardial Revascularization

An investigational procedure termed transmyocardial revascularization is currently undergoing a clinical trial. As performed on patients who are not suited for standard revascularization procedures, a laser creates a channel in the ischemic regions of the myocardium. These laser-made holes or channels allow interventricular blood to perfuse the myocardium in a manner similar to reptilian myocardial perfusion. Currently the technique requires a thoracotomy, but in the future it may be possible for the laser surgery to be performed via a heart catheter similar to the current catheter-ablation techniques for accessory conduction pathways.

Exercise Training

Regular physical activity may improve exercise-related myocardial is-chemia (Squires 1995). After a period of exercise training, for a specific submaximal exercise intensity the myocardial oxygen requirement, as indicated by the product of heart rate and systolic blood pressure (the rate-pressure product), is reduced (see figure 2.2).

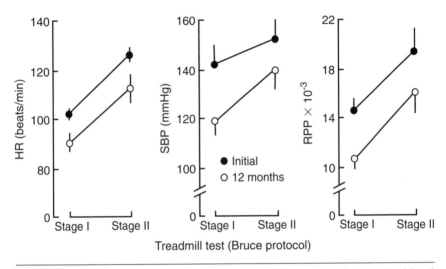

Figure 2.2   Effects of exercise training on heart rate (HR), systolic blood pressure (SBP), and rate-pressure product (RPP) at stages I and II of the Bruce treadmill protocol. All variables, after 12 months of training, were significantly lower ($p < .01$) than before training.

Reprinted from *The American Journal of Cardiology*, 50, Ehsani AA, Martin WH, Heath GW, Coyle EF., Cardiac effects of prolonged and intense exercise training in patients with coronary artery disease, 249, Copyright 1982, with permission from Excerpta Medica Inc.

After exercise training, the patient may perform more intense physical activity before exceeding the ischemic threshold (the rate-pressure product that corresponds to the onset of ischemia). In addition, there is evidence that for some patients the rate-pressure product at the ischemic threshold is increased by training independent of alterations in anti-ischemic drug therapy, suggesting that myocardial blood flow may be improved (Raffo et al. 1980; Laslett et al. 1985).

Thallium myocardial perfusion during graded exercise before and after a period of exercise training has, in selected patients, demonstrated im-proved myocardial perfusion. Reductions in exercise-induced ischemia of

54% and 34% at maximal exercise intensities measured by thallium perfusion have been reported (Schuler et al. 1988; Todd et al. 1991). Although there are no angiographic data to support the concept of development of coronary collateral vessels with exercise training (Franklin 1991; Niebauer et al. 1995), the thallium defect improvement with habitual exercise suggests either improved blood rheology (decreased viscosity) or improved regional blood flow through the previously ischemic myocardium. Preliminary data suggest that pretreatment (20 to 30 minutes before exercise training) with heparin may augment the effect of exercise training on lessening ischemia (Gagliardi et al. 1996). Heparin may stimulate collateral circulation development in the setting of myocardial ischemia.

Exercise training, in sufficient quantities, appears to retard the progression or reverse coronary atherosclerosis (Hambrecht et al. 1993). In a randomized study, 60 patients with definite coronary atherosclerosis received quantitative coronary angiography before and after one year of exercise training or control conditions. All patients were instructed in a low-fat, low-cholesterol diet, and medications were held constant. Angiographic progression of disease occurred in 45% of controls and 10% of exercisers. No change in lesion appearance was observed in 62% of exercisers compared with 49% of controls. Regression of atherosclerosis was observed in 28% of exercisers versus 6% of controls. Regression of disease was observed only in patients who expended an average of 2,200 kilocalories per week in physical activity, which required approximately five to six hours of moderate exercise training per week.

Risk Factor Reduction

Aggressive control of the risk factors of cigarette smoking, hypertension, dyslipidemia, obesity, high-fat diet, and psychosocial stress has an important place in the treatment of coronary artery disease in patients with and without evidence of myocardial ischemia (Squires et al. 1996).

Smoking

Smoking causes the displacement of oxygen from hemoglobin by carbon monoxide, thus reducing the arterial oxygen content. Nicotine from smoke is a potent vasoconstrictor and platelet activator. All patients with ischemia must stop the use of all tobacco products.

Hypertension

Elevated blood pressure increases myocardial oxygen requirement and may provoke or increase the severity of ischemia.

Obesity

Obesity increases myocardial work and leads to left ventricular hypertrophy, hypertension, and insulin resistance with associated blood platelet abnormalities and an adverse blood lipid profile. A diet high in kilocalories, total fat, saturated fat, and cholesterol may result in dyslipidemia, obesity, insulin resistance, hypertension, and progression of atherosclerosis (Kottke et al. 1996).

Stress

Emotional stress may trigger myocardial ischemia, myocardial infarction, and sudden cardiac death. Leor and colleagues (1996) examined records of the Department of Coroner of Los Angeles County around the time period of January 17, 1994, the date of a major earthquake centered near Northridge, California. Figure 2.3 displays the abrupt increase in definite sudden cardiac deaths on the day of the earthquake. Only three of the 24 deaths occurred during or immediately after heavy physical exertion. A 35% increase in hospitalizations for acute myocardial infarction in the 72 coronary care units in southern California was observed in the week after the earthquake (Leor and Kloner 1995). An increase in the number of implantable cardioverter-defibrillator discharges during the two-week period after the earthquake was also reported (Nishimoto et al. 1995).

Presumably, stress-mediated release of catecholamines and hypercoagulability factors contributed to plaque rupture and subsequent thrombosis, as well as to ventricular arrhythmias.

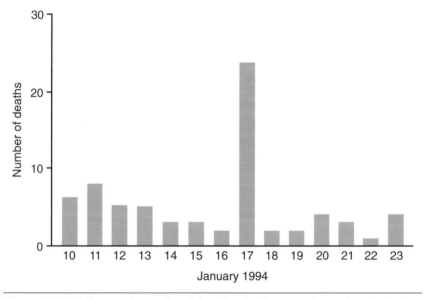

Figure 2.3   Daily numbers of sudden deaths due to atherosclerosis in Los Angeles County in January 1994. On January 17, the day of the Northridge earthquake, 24 cases of sudden death were reported (p < .01 vs. other days).

Psychosocial interventions such as stress management, relaxation therapy, group or individual psychotherapy, and type A behavior counseling will lessen psychological distress and lower systolic blood pressure, heart rate, serum cholesterol, cardiac mortality, and recurrent myocardial infarction (Linden et al. 1996). For patients with demonstrable myocardial ischemia with signs of severe time urgency and hostility (two components of type A behavior), specific type A behavioral counseling reduces ambulatory ECG ischemic episode frequency (Friedman et al. 1996). Transcendental meditation has been shown to reduce exercise test-related myocardial ischemia (delayed onset of ST segment depression) and improve exercise tolerance without systematic exercise training or additional anti-ischemic medications (Zamarra et al. 1996).

Blood Lipids

An adverse blood lipid profile (elevated low-density lipoprotein cholesterol, low levels of high-density lipoprotein cholesterol, elevated triglycerides) is an indisputable major risk factor for coronary atherosclerosis. In addition to its obvious role in the development of obstructive coronary atherosclerotic lesions, hypercholesterolemia results in impaired endothelial-dependent and endothelial-independent relaxation of small coronary arteries (Goode and Heagerty 1995; Henry et al. 1995). This impairment of vasomotion causes exercise-related myocardial ischemia in some patients (Zeiher et al. 1995).

Reducing elevated blood cholesterol concentrations restores endothelium-dependent vasodilation (Egashira et al. 1994; Treasure et al. 1995). Furthermore, some lesions, because of their anatomic features, are prone to rupture, with subsequent platelet thrombus formation resulting in increased lesion bulk (Chesebro et al. 1991; Falk et al. 1995). This lesion rupture may lead to the development of unstable angina, acute myocardial infarction, and sudden cardiac death. Elevated blood cholesterol concentrations increase the potential for thrombogenesis, as well. Cholesterol lowering may stabilize rupture-prone lesions and reduce thrombogenesis.

Angiographic trials of lipid lowering in patients with coronary atherosclerosis by means of very low-fat diets, medications, or partial ileal bypass surgery have shown consistently that, in the time frame of only a few years, lesion progression is slowed, regression of disease occurs in some patients, fewer cardiac events occur, and cardiovascular and total mortality are lower in treated patients than in controls (Blankenhorn et al. 1987; Buchwald et al. 1992; Gotto 1995; Gould 1994; Ornish et al. 1990; Waters et al. 1995). The Scandinavian Simvastatin Survival Study Group (1994) demonstrated a reduced relative risk of death of 0.58 compared to controls with aggressive cholesterol lowering. Nonfatal myocardial infarctions, resuscitated sudden death, the need for revascularization, and cerebrovascular events were lower in the treatment group.

The magnitude of the angiographic improvement reported in the regression trials was minimal, an average of 1% to 3% improvement in luminal caliber, but the reduction in clinical events was 25% to 75% (Topol and Nissen 1995).

After lowering lipids, a reduction in myocardial ischemia at rest and dipyridamole stress images has been reported by positron emission tomography (Gould et al. 1995). Lowering cholesterol also reduces the myocardial ischemia of daily life assessed with ambulatory ECGs (Andrews et al. 1997), as well as exercise-induced ischemia assessed with graded exercise testing (de Divitiis et al. 1996). Cholesterol lowering also corrects exercise-related abnormal coronary vasoconstriction and reduces thrombogenecity (Seiler et al. 1995).

The improvement in clinical outcomes for patients receiving lipid-lowering therapy may, in part, be due to regression of some lesions, but is also due to stabilization of lesions leading to less plaque rupture and thrombosis (Stark 1996). The Adult Treatment Panel II guidelines from the National Cholesterol Education Program (Expert Panel on Detection, Evaluation, and Treatment of High Blood Cholesterol in Adults 1993) reflect the growing body of convincing evidence regarding the benefits of aggressive blood lipid management in patients with atherosclerosis.

The recommended low-density lipoprotein cholesterol (LDL-C) concentration for patients with disease is less than or equal to 100 mg/dl. This goal may be achieved in most patients with coronary artery disease using a combination of the lifestyle factors of a very low-fat diet, exercise training, body fat loss, and prudent use of lipid-level improving medications such as HMG Co-A reductase inhibitors, nicotinic acid, gemfibrozil, and cholestyramine.

Diets extremely low in total and saturated fat and cholesterol have been shown to be effective in reducing LDL-C and slowing or reversing coronary atherosclerosis (Ornish et al. 1990). In addition, a Mediterranean-type diet (containing omega-3 fatty acids, oleic acid, and antioxidant vitamins), while not low in total fat, has been demonstrated to reduce cardiovascular deaths, nonfatal myocardial infarction, total mortality, development of unstable angina, and elective myocardial revascularization. (de Lorgeril et al. 1996).

Left Ventricular Dysfunction and Chronic Heart Failure

As the population ages, the prevalence of chronic heart failure, which currently affects 4.7 million Americans, and its incidence, presently 400,000 new cases per year with 900,000 hospitalizations annually, will increase (Cardiology Preeminence Roundtable 1994). This is a result of the increasing prevalence and cumulative duration of hypertension and coronary artery disease with advancing age (Senni and Redfield 1997). Chronic heart failure is the only major cardiovascular disease with an increasing prevalence and incidence. Heart failure prevalence of 1% in persons aged 50 to 59 years increases to 10% for octogenarians (Duncan et al. 1996). Currently, 13% of the population of the United States is over 65 years of age; 21% of the population will be over 65 by the year 2030 (Redfield 1996). Chronic heart failure is the most common diagnostic-related group classification for hospitalized Medicare patients, at an estimated cost of $3.1 billion in 1991. Total direct health care costs for all patients with chronic heart failure is approximately $18 billion each year (Cohn et al. 1997). Unfortunately, chronic heart failure is also an all-too-common syndrome in younger patients. For example, population estimates of the prevalence of idiopathic dilated cardiomyopathy in persons less than 55 years of age is 18 per 100,000 population (Codd et al. 1989). Chronic heart failure is a highly lethal condition.

The most common causes of left ventricular systolic and diastolic dysfunction are the following (Karon 1995; American College of Cardiology/American Heart Association Task Force Report 1995):

- Coronary artery disease
- Idiopathic dilated cardiomyopathy
- Hypertension

Additional diseases that may potentially result in chronic heart failure include valvular heart disease, myocarditis, alcohol abuse, chemotherapy, acquired immunodeficiency syndrome, infiltrative diseases of the myocardium, pericardial disease, peripartum, muscular dystrophy, tachycardia, and pheochromocytoma.

Diagnosis of Chronic Heart Failure

Systolic dysfunction results in poor contractile performance and is commonly diagnosed by a below normal left ventricular ejection fraction (<50% as measured by echocardiography, radionuclide ventriculography, etc.).

Diastolic dysfunction is the condition in which the heart cannot accept blood and fill at a normal diastolic pressure, and results in inadequate left ventricular filling, slow filling, or the development of abnormally high ventricular diastolic pressure. Hypertension is a common cause of chronic heart failure in the elderly as a result of left ventricular hypertrophy and fibrosis, endothelial dysfunction and coronary microvascular disease. Diastolic dysfunction is diagnosed by abnormal echo Doppler patterns of relaxation and compliance, and catheterization evidence of increased left ventricular filling pressures without evidence of systolic dysfunction.

Some patients have either predominantly systolic or diastolic dysfunction, while others have both conditions concurrently. Either systolic or diastolic dysfunction may result in symptomatic chronic heart failure. Cardiac output and blood pressure may be inadequate for tissue oxygenation in chronic heart failure, and fluid overload (congestion) and reduced exercise tolerance may develop (Gaasch 1994; Karon 1995; Packer 1990; Vasan et al. 1995).

Pulmonary hypertension is frequent in patients with left ventricular dysfunction, but pulmonary artery systolic pressures vary widely, are independent of ejection fraction, and are positively associated with diastolic dysfunction (Enriquez-Sarano et al. 1997).

Progression of Chronic Heart Failure

The natural history of chronic heart failure usually includes a variable period of time with an asymptomatic stage of depressed left ventricular ejection fraction with cardiomegally (asymptomatic left ventricular dysfunction). This progresses to a minimally symptomatic stage and finally to the stage of congestive symptoms. The rate of deterioration is highly variable (Rodeheffer and Gersh 1996). Symptoms that commonly develop in patients with chronic heart failure include the following:

- Fatigue, weakness
- Dyspnea, especially with exertion
- Reduced exercise capacity
- Orthopnea or paroxysmal nocturnal dyspnea

Compared with healthy subjects, some patients with stable, severe heart failure develop impaired cognitive brain function (Grimm et al. 1996). This is probably a result of a reduced oxygen and nutrient supply to the brain secondary to an inadequate cardiac output. However, many patients have a moderate to severe reduction in left ventricular ejection fraction and remain minimally symptomatic or even asymptomatic due to compensatory physiological adaptations that will be discussed later in the chapter.

The term congestive heart failure is reserved for patients with evidence of fluid overload, while the terms chronic heart failure or left ventricular dysfunction describe patients with cardiac function impairment who may or may not have signs or symptoms of congestion. In left heart failure, congestion occurs in the pulmonary circulation, while in right heart failure fluid overload is located in the peripheral tissues. Biventricular failure may result in both pulmonary and peripheral congestion.

Once symptoms of congestive failure develop, median survival is only 2-3 years. In the Framingham study, six-year mortality was 80% and 65% for men and women, respectively (Kannel and Belanger 1991). Mortality is higher with increasing age, and many patients with heart failure are over 65 years of age and have significant additional comorbidities. Asymptomatic left ventricular dysfunction is associated with a two-year mortality of 10%

to 15% (Redfield 1996); seven-year mortality is approximately 50% (Redfield et al. 1994). With improved detection and treatment with angiotensin-converting enzyme inhibitors in recent years, there is evidence that mortality is improving (see figure 2.4).

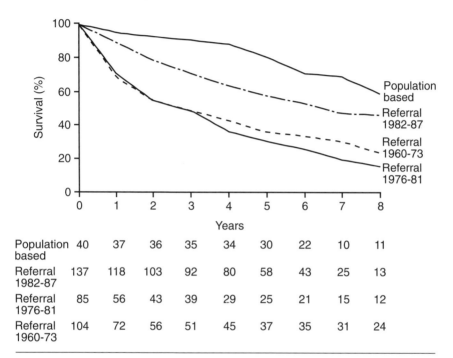

	0	1	2	3	4	5	6	7	8
Population based	40	37	36	35	34	30	22	10	11
Referral 1982-87	137	118	103	92	80	58	43	25	13
Referral 1976-81	85	56	43	39	29	25	21	15	12
Referral 1960-73	104	72	56	51	45	37	35	31	24

Figure 2.4   Survival curves for four cohorts of patients with idiopathic dilated cardiomyopathy. Survival in the 1976-1981 and 1960-1973 referral cohorts was similar. Survival in the 1982-1987 referral cohort was better than for the two earlier referral cohorts, but not as favorable as for the population-based cohort.

Reprinted from *Journal of the American College of Cardiology*, 22, Redfield MM, Gersh BJ, Baily KR, Ballard DJ, Rodeheffer RJ., Natural history of idiopathic dilated cardiomyopathy: Effect of referral bias and secular trend, 1924, Copyright 1993, with permission from the American College of Cardiology.

Some conditions leading to left ventricular dysfunction such as alcohol abuse, valvular heart disease, myocardial ischemia, and tachycardia are potentially reversed by treatment. However, irrespective of etiology, the results of chronic heart failure in terms of symptoms and outcome are remarkably similar.

Compensatory Physiology in Chronic Heart Failure

Cardiac and extracardiac physiological compensatory adjustments are activated when left ventricular function is depressed (Rodeheffer et al.

1996). These compensatory adaptations are designed to maintain an adequate cardiac output for tissue perfusion and are beneficial in the short term (days to weeks). However, in chronic left ventricular dysfunction, these adjustments may actually contribute to progressive ventricular and vascular dysfunction, ultimately resulting in severe congestive heart failure.

Cardiac Adjustments

Cardiac adjustments to depressed left ventricular function include left ventricular dilatation and concentric hypertrophy resulting in an increased end-diastolic volume and augmented stroke volume via the Frank-Starling mechanism (Cohn 1995). With contractile dysfunction, ventricular remodeling occurs as a result of myocyte loss, interstitial fibrosis, myocardial slippage, and myocyte hypertrophy (Francis et al. 1995), which results in progressive dilatation and hypertrophy of the cardiac chambers. End-diastolic volume enlarges to maintain stroke volume in the setting of a reduced left ventricular ejection fraction. An increase in heart rate also occurs, due to increased sympathetic nervous system activity, to help maintain cardiac output.

Over time, additional ventricular dilatation and hypertrophy may occur in response to increased wall stress, which leads to further deterioration in systolic function. Increased passive ventricular wall stiffness and slowed energy-dependent myocyte relaxation result in further diastolic dysfunction. There is evidence that the failing heart has an impaired ability to regenerate the high-energy phosphate compounds necessary for adequate contractile function (Katz 1993).

Substances such as endothelin (Wei et al. 1994) and angiotensin II (Raman et al. 1995) have been implicated as direct agents responsible for cardiac hypertrophy and fibrosis in heart failure.

Tumor necrosis factor and interleukin-6, cytokines produced by inflammatory cells, are increased in patients with congestive heart failure and result in cachexia (profound loss of lean body mass, anorexia, malnutrition, and inflammation), marked activation of the renin-angiotensin-aldosterone system, left ventricular dysfunction, and pulmonary edema (Packer 1995; Ferrari et al. 1995; Torre-Amione et al. 1996a; Torre-Amione et al. 1996b). Blood ketone bodies may be elevated due to increased free fatty acid mobilization in response to neurohormonal stimulation (Lommi et al. 1996).

Extracardiac Adjustments

Activation of the sympathetic nervous system and the renin-angiotensin-aldosterone system is the primary extracardiac compensatory mechanism for depressed left ventricular function (Benedict et al. 1994; Kaye et al. 1995). The result is peripheral vasoconstriction mediated by direct sympathetic nervous system effects on the vasculature as well as by hormones such as the catecholamines, angiotensin II, endothelin, and arginine vasopressin

(Demopoulos and LeJemtel 1994; Krum et al. 1995a). Changes in regional circulations occur, that result in preservation of blood flow to the brain and heart at the expense of the renal, skeletal muscle, splanchnic, and cutaneous circulations.

Sodium and water retention by the kidney cause an increase in blood volume. The increase in vascular resistance and blood volume may be adequate to maintain blood pressure and the patient may be well compensated and asymptomatic. However, if these neural and hormonal adjustments are inadequate to maintain cardiac output, or if over time the neurohormonal activation worsens cardiac function, decompensation occurs and the patient develops progressive symptoms such as fatigue, dyspnea on exertion, a profoundly reduced exercise tolerance, orthopnia, paroxysmal nocturnal dyspnea, edema, and even cardiogenic shock. The New York Heart Association classification of heart failure symptom severity (see table 2.1) is used to grade the symptomatic status of patients (Goldman et al. 1981).

Table 2.1   New York Heart Association Functional Classification

Class I	Patients with cardiac disease but without resulting limitations of physical activity. Ordinary physical activity does not cause undue fatigue, palpitation, dyspnea, or anginal pain.
Class II	Patients with cardiac disease resulting in slight limitation of physical activity. They are comfortable at rest. Ordinary physical activity results in fatigue, palpitation, dyspnea, or anginal pain.
Class III	Patients with cardiac disease resulting in marked limitation of physical activity. They are comfortable at rest. Less than ordinary physical activity causes fatigue, palpitations, dyspnea, or angina pain.
Class IV	Patients with cardiac disease resulting in inability to carry on any physical activity without discomfort. Symptoms of cardiac insufficiency or of the anginal syndrome may be present even at rest. If any physical activity is undertaken, discomfort is increased.

Reproduced, with permission, from Goldman L, Hashimoto B, Cook EF, Loscalzo A. Comparative reproducibility and validity of systems for assessing cardiovascular functional class: advantages of a new specific activity scale. *Circulation* 64:1228. Copyright 1981 American Heart Association.

Cellular changes, such as desensitization of beta receptors and atrial baroreceptors, and skeletal muscle abnormalities also occur (Rodeheffer et al. 1996; Grassi et al. 1995). The down-regulation of beta receptors functions to protect the heart from catecholamine toxicity. However, baroreceptor dysfunction results in reduced diuresis, and may lead to excessive fluid retention and increased left atrial pressure.

As a result of neurohormonal activation and, in part, to inactivity, skeletal muscle abnormalities occur, such as reduction in aerobic metabolic enzyme activity, and transformation from type I (slow twitch) to type II (fast twitch) motor unit physiology (Massie et al. 1996). Some of these changes are similar to the normal aging process (Trappe et al. 1995) or deconditioning, although the degree of alteration is often extreme in chronic heart failure. Due to excessive vessel wall stiffness and endothelial dysfunction, skeletal muscle vasodilatation is impaired, which further reduces muscle perfusion and exercise capacity (Demopoulos and LeJemtel 1994). Respiratory muscle strength and endurance is also impaired in heart failure (Evans et al. 1995; Mancini et al. 1994).

The physiology of oxygen transport and delivery by the blood is also altered in patients with severe left ventricular dysfunction. Arterial oxygen content, probably related to renal hypoperfusion-mediated excess erythro-poietin release, is increased in patients with moderate heart failure (Herrlin and Sylven 1991). Increased 2,3-DPG concentration, which favors oxygen unloading from the capillary blood at the tissue level, has also been reported in these patients (Bersin et al. 1993). These two adjustments are additional examples of physiological compensation to maintain tissue oxygenation in the face of left ventricular dysfunction.

A behavioral compensation occurs in some patients as a result of their symptoms of left ventricular dysfunction. In patients with heart failure of a degree sufficient to warrant listing for cardiac transplantation, the most common symptoms include tiredness, difficulty breathing during physical activity, difficulty sleeping, weakness, and sleepiness (Grady et al. 1992). In order to minimize symptoms, patients with heart failure often self-restrict physical activity. Oka and colleagues (1993) studied daily physical activity by use of a heart rate monitor in 45 patients and determined that activity levels were low and were out of proportion to the patients' measured exercise capacities. Deconditioning, exacerbated by inactivity, will worsen symptoms and probably cause an even further decrease in spontaneous physical activity.

Chronic heart failure is said to be compensated if the physiological responses to left ventricular dysfunction discussed above are adequate to maintain cardiac output and blood pressure. If there is a progressive decrease in cardiac output and blood pressure despite activation of physiological systems (leading to vasoconstriction and fluid retention), the heart failure is termed uncompensated with resultant congestive signs and symptoms.

Treatment of Chronic Heart Failure

The treatment of patients with ventricular dysfunction may include medications, lifestyle changes or improvements, and surgery (American College of Cardiology/American Heart Association Task Force Report 1995; Agency for Health Care Policy and Research 1994; Olson and Miller 1996; Karon 1995; Massie 1994). Cardiac rehabilitation services should be considered an integral part of optimal patient management.

Medical Treatment

The following classes of medications play important roles in the treatment of chronic heart failure:

- Diuretics
- Angiotensin-converting enzyme (ACE) inhibitors
- Positive inotropic agents (digoxin, dobutamine)
- Nitrates
- Vasodilators (hydralazine)
- Beta blockers
- Calcium channel blockers
- Anticoagulants
- Blood lipid improving agents

Drugs that improve dyslipidemia have an important positive effect on patients with coronary atherosclerosis and were discussed previously in this chapter.

Diuretics

Diuretics are essential for the control of edema in patients with fluid volume overload and symptoms of pulmonary and systemic congestion.

ACE Inhibitors

ACE inhibitors are indicated for all patients with left ventricular dysfunction unless the patient cannot tolerate them or exhibits a contraindication for their use such as hypotension, high-renin states, over-diuresis, or significant renal failure (Opie 1995). ACE inhibitors prevent or slow the progression of asymptomatic left ventricular dysfunction to congestive failure and forestall adverse ventricular remodeling. These drugs also reduce hospitalization rates and mortality, reduce symptoms of heart failure, potentially increase exercise tolerance, and improve patient quality of life (Cleland 1994; Garg and Yusuf 1995; Greenberg et al. 1995; Mancini et al. 1987; Rogers et al. 1994). These agents are the only available treatment, other than transplantation, that have been demonstrated to improve survival for all classes of heart failure. The following clinical trials of ACE inhibitors have reported benefits for patients with symptoms:

- Veterans Administration heart failure trial (V-Heft II)
- Studies of left ventricular dysfunction (SOLVD)
- Cooperative north Scandinavian enalapril survival study (CONSEN-SUS)

The following additional trials have been performed in asymptomatic patients and have demonstrated a survival benefit:

- Survival and ventricular enlargement trial (SAVE)
- SOLVD prevention arm
- Munich mild heart failure trial

Recently, angiotensin II receptor blockers have become available and are currently under investigation for use in heart failure (Dickstein et al. 1995). This class of drug may be extremely helpful for patients who cannot take ACE inhibitors.

Digoxin

Digoxin improves cardiac output and exercise capacity in heart failure patients, reduces left ventricular end-diastolic pressure, may reduce heart size, and decreases pulmonary and systemic congestion as well (Sullivan et al. 1989). It is useful for patients with chronic heart failure who also have atrial fibrillation.

Dobutamine

For patients with intractable congestive failure, infusions of dobutamine during hospitalization or on an outpatient basis may be helpful in reducing symptoms and improving exercise capacity (Erlemeier et al. 1992).

Nitrates and Hydralazine

Nitrates and hydralazine improve symptoms in heart failure patients, improve survival in class II-III patients, and are an important alternative for patients who cannot tolerate ACE inhibitors (Olson and Miller 1996).

Beta Blockers

Beta blockers such as metoprolol and bucindolol, while considered experimental for the treatment of chronic heart failure, improve left ventricular function and exercise hemodynamics in patients with either ischemic left ventricular dysfunction or idiopathic dilated cardiomyopathy (Andersson et al. 1994; Bristow et al. 1994; Krum et al. 1995b).

Neurohormonal activation in the failing heart leads to the long-term consequences of progressive myocardial dysfunction. In addition to angiotensin-converting enzyme inhibition, investigators have recently evaluated beta adrenergic receptor blockers in patients with chronic heart failure. In particular, carvedilol (a nonselective beta blocker with alpha receptor blocking effects and antioxidant properties) has been shown to decrease mortality and the need for hospitalization, increase left ventricular ejection fraction, and improve symptoms (Packer et al. 1996a; Packer et al. 1996b). Although carvedilol treatment does not apparently improve exercise tolerance in CHF (Bristow et al. 1996), it does retard the usual progressive deterioration in left ventricular function (Eichhorn and Bristow 1996). Benefits have been reported for patients who are only mildly symptomatic, as well (Colucci et al. 1996). Carvedilol recently received FDA approval for patients with mild to moderate (NYHA class II or III) heart failure.

Investigational Medical Therapy
Some additional medical therapies are under investigation and may prove to be clinically important in the future. Pimobendan, a phosphodiesterase inhibitor with positive inotropic and vasodilating properties, has been shown to improve exercise capacity, although a trend for increased mortality was noted in a recent clinical trial (The Pimobendan in Congestive Heart Failure [PICO] Investigators 1996). L-thyroxine treatment for three months in patients with idiopathic dilated cardiomyopathy demonstrated a modest increase in ejection fraction, peak exercise cardiac output, and exercise capacity (Moruzzi et al. 1996). L-arginine supplementation, which theoretically should increase the amount of the vasodilator nitric oxide, was demonstrated to increase forearm blood flow during exercise as well as increase the six-minute walk distance in CHF patients (Rector et al. 1996). For CHF patients who exhibit Cheynne-Stokes respiration during sleep with repetitive oxygen desaturation and impaired sleep, nocturnal nasal supplemental oxygen improves sleep, exercise capacity, and cognitive function (Andreas et al. 1996).

Drug Treatment of Diastolic Dysfunction
Drug treatment for patients with isolated diastolic dysfunction includes the use of beta and calcium channel blockers to reduce heart rate and increase diastolic filling time (Olson and Miller 1996). ACE inhibitors may also be given to promote ventricular filling at lower atrial pressures. Filling pressures may also be reduced with the use of diuretics and nitrates.

Treatment of Ventricular Arrhythmias
Many patients with chronic heart failure have ventricular arrhythmias. Arrhythmic sudden cardiac death ultimately is responsible for the demise of 40% to 50% of heart failure patients (Olson and Miller 1996). In general, asymptomatic arrhythmias do not require pharmacological treatment. Symptomatic ventricular arrhythmias require treatment tailored to the patient, and may consist of improved treatment of ventricular failure,

electrophysiological testing of directed antiarrhythmic medications such as beta blockers or amiodarone, treatment of underlying myocardial ischemia with drugs or revascularization, or placement of an implantable cardioverter-defibrillator (Batsford et al. 1995). The recently published multicenter automatic defibrillator implantation trial (MADIT) demonstrated that prophylactic therapy with an implanted cardioverter-defibrillator, compared with conventional medical therapy, improved survival in postmyocardial infarction patients with left ventricular dysfunction and nonsustained ventricular tachycardia (Moss et al. 1996).

Anticoagulation Medications

Patients with heart failure are at increased risk for venous and arterial thromboembolism. Some clinicians recommend prophylactic anticoagulation for patients with a dilated left ventricle and LVEF < 35%. All patients with left ventricular dysfunction and atrial fibrillation should receive anticoagulation (Olson and Miller 1996). Antithrombotic therapy with either antiplatelet or anticoagulant agents has been shown to reduce the risk of sudden cardiac death in patients with CHF (Dries et al. 1997).

Psychological Factors

Emotional distress, anxiety, and depression are prevalent in patients with symptomatic heart failure (Soler-Soler and Permanyer-Miralda 1994). Appropriate psychiatric care should be provided. However, many patients who do not require treatment by a psychiatrist do benefit from supportive care and education. Support group activities for patients and families are particularly beneficial and economical.

Lifestyle Factors

Lifestyle factors, including diet, smoking cessation, exercise training, and stress management activities, are critical in reducing risk.

Dietary Factors

Dietary sodium restriction to < 3 gm/day for most patients and < 2 gm/day for patients with severe edema is extremely important (Karon 1995). Daily body weight measurements may alert patients of insidious fluid weight gain. Avoidance of alcohol, a negative intropic substance, is recommended. Fluid intake restriction is recommended for patients with congestive signs or symptoms.

A low-fat/low-cholesterol diet is important for patients with either obesity or atherosclerosis. Correction of obesity is an important treatment goal.

Some patients with chronic heart failure have thiamin deficiency, which may result in worsening biventricular failure and fluid retention (Brady et al. 1995). Thiamin supplementation has been shown to improve left ventricular systolic function in some patients (Shimon et al. 1995).

Smoking

Cigarette smoke reduces the oxygen-carrying capacity of the blood, promotes vasoconstriction, and is atherogenic (Soler-Soler and Permanyer-Miralda 1994; Squires and Williams 1993). Patients must give high priority to complete avoidance of tobacco.

Exercise Training

Exercise training, for properly selected patients, improves exercise tolerance. Unless specifically contraindicated, an exercise program should be considered an integral part of the treatment of every heart failure patient. Chapters 4 and 5 provide a complete description of the benefits and techniques of exercise training for patients with chronic heart failure. Specific respiratory muscle training may be indicated for patients with respiratory muscle weakness.

Patient and Family Education

Patients with heart failure are required to make significant adjustments in their lifestyles including taking medications per schedule, restricting dietary intake, avoiding tobacco, exercise training, and potentially restricting some physical activities associated with occupation or avocation. Noncompliance may lead to unnecessary hospitalizations, physician office visits, or early death. Careful patient and family education and counseling have been demonstrated to improve patient compliance and outcomes as well as decrease hospitalizations (Dracup et al. 1994).

Patient and family education for chronic heart failure may include the following topics:

- Heart failure pathophysiology
- Lifestyle modification
- Monitoring medical therapy
- Common diagnostic procedures
- Medications
- Pacemakers
- Cardiac transplantation
- Cardioversion

Resources for patient and family education regarding chronic heart failure are numerous. The following list includes a few good sources of information.

U.S. Department of Health and Human Services; Public Health Service; Agency for Health Care Policy and Research. *Clinical Practice Guideline Number 11: Heart Failure Management of Patients with Left-Ventricular Systolic Dysfunction.* AHCPR Publication No. 94-0613. Washington, DC: U.S. Government Printing Office. 1994. Telephone (202) 512-1800.

This comprehensive document includes patient counseling information including the definition, diagnosis, causes, and prognosis of chronic heart failure; symptoms of worsening heart failure and appropriate patient responses to symptoms; physical activity, diet, medications, and compliance issues; and information on the health care team.

> Dibianco R. *You Can Live with Heart Failure: What You Can Do to Live a Better, More Comfortable Life.* E.R. Squibb and Sons. Princeton, NJ. 1991. Available from Squibb.

This is a comprehensive patient education booklet (68 pages) covering the definition and causes of chronic heart failure; diet, rest, exercise, and sexual activity; and medications and tests used in chronic heart failure.

> American Heart Association. *Congestive Heart Failure: What You Should Know.* American Heart Association National Center, 7272 Greenville Avenue, Dallas, TX 75231-4596.

This 12-page pamphlet provides basic information regarding chronic heart failure causes, pathophysiology, signs and symptoms, and exercise and treatment options.

> *Heart Failure: What You Should Know.* Merck and Co. 1996. Available from Merck.

This concise pamphlet (13 pages) provides the definition of chronic heart failure and discusses symptoms, diagnostic tests, treatment options, medications, and lifestyle factors.

> *Living Successfully with Heart Failure: Changes You Can Make for a Healthier Heart . . . One Step at a Time.* Bristol-Myers Squibb Co. Princeton, NJ 08543. 1996. Available from Bristol-Myers Squibb.

This is a brief pamphlet (14 pages) with a behavioral modification approach to topics that include the following:

- Chronic heart failure pathophysiology, symptoms
- Medications
- Questions frequently asked about CHF
- Lifestyle factors—diet, smoking cessation, exercise, rest
- Setting goals
- Records—daily weights, symptoms, weekly goals, questions for the doctor

▌ *Congestive Heart Failure.* Kramer Communications. 1992. Telephone (800) ▌ 333-3032.

This is a well-illustrated booklet (15 pages) covering these topics: definition and causes of chronic heart failure; warning symptoms, heart evaluations, treatment plans and medications; diet, rest, and physical activity.

For patients with symptoms of fatigue and dyspnea that make activities of daily living difficult, an occupational therapist consultation concerning energy saving is helpful. Common tips taught to CHF patients by occupational therapists include the following:

- Avoid rushing through tasks
- Rest before you become tired
- Relax between tasks
- Slide objects rather than lift them
- Don't hold objects for a prolonged time
- Sit to reduce energy expenditure during repetitive tasks
- Delegate tiring work to others

Rich and associates (1995) conducted a randomized trial to assess the effectiveness of a nurse-directed, multidisciplinary intervention on hospital readmission rates and treatment costs for 282 patients (142 in the treatment group, 140 controls) over 70 years of age with a recent hospitalization for congestive heart failure. The intervention consisted of the following components:

- Education of patient and family by a cardiovascular nurse
- Individualized dietary consultation and recommendations by a registered dietitian
- Discharge planning with social service personnel
- Analysis and simplification of the drug regimen for each patient by a geriatric cardiologist
- Intensive follow-up via the hospital's home care service, individualized home visits, and telephone calls from members of the study team

Survival for 90 days tended to be better for treatment patients (91 of 142 patients for the treatment group; 75 of 140 patients in the control group, p = .09). There were significantly fewer hospital readmissions for the treatment group compared with the controls, 53 versus 94, respectively. Overall cost of medical care was $460 less for treatment patients versus control patients. Cardiac rehabilitation programs could provide much of this type of patient education and follow-up.

Surgery

Surgical revascularization with catheter-based techniques or coronary bypass surgery plays an important role in preventing further ischemic injury and may restore hibernating myocardium and thus improve left ventricular function in patients with coronary artery disease (Magovern et al. 1993).

Cardiac transplantation is the accepted treatment of choice for appropriate patients with end-stage heart failure. Experimental surgical techniques, including implantation of left ventricular assist devices and cardiomyoplasty, are currently under evaluation (Moreira et al. 1991). Some patients with dilated cardiomyopathy may show hemodynamic benefit from dual chamber pacing (Nishimura et al. 1996). Pacing appears to benefit some patients with prolonged atrioventricular conduction by restoring appropriate atrioventricular synchrony. Surgical removal of a wedge of the left ventricle (partial left ventriculectomy) in order to reduce heart size and increase ejection fraction in patients with end-stage cardiomyopathy not considered candidates for transplantation is currently under investigation. Preliminary results are encouraging.

In summary, the pathophysiology of myocardial ischemia and chronic heart failure is well established as outlined in this chapter. Treatment options for patients include medications, surgery, and lifestyle modifications including exercise training.

References

U.S. Department of Health and Human Services; Public Health Service; Agency for Health Care Policy and Research. 1994. *Clinical Practice Guideline Number 11: Heart Failure Management of Patients with Left-Ventricular Systolic Dysfunction.* (AHCPR Publication No. 94-0613). Washington, DC: U.S. Government Printing Office.

American College of Cardiology/American Heart Association Task Force Report. 1995. Guidelines for the evaluation and management of heart failure: Report of the American College of Cardiology/American Heart Association task force on practice guidelines committee on evaluation and management of heart failure. *J Am Coll Cardiol* 26:1376-1398.

Andersson B, Hamm C, Persson S, Wikstrom G, Sinagra G, Hjalmarson A, Waagstein F. 1994. Improved exercise hemodynamic status in dilated cardiomyopathy after beta adrenergic blockade treatment. *J Am Coll Cardiol* 23:1397-1404.

Andreas S, Clemens C, Sandholzer H, Figulla HR, Kreuzer H. 1996. Improvement of exercise capacity with treatment of Cheyne-Stokes respiration in patients with congestive heart failure. *J Am Coll Cardiol* 27:1486-1490.

Andrews TC, Raby K, Barry J, Naimi CL, Allred E, Ganz P, Selwyn AP.

1997. Effect of cholesterol reduction on myocardial ischemia in patients with coronary disease. *Circulation* 95:324-328.

Batsford WP, Mickleborough LL, Elefteriades JA. 1995. Ventricular arrhythmias in heart failure. *Cardiol Clin* 13:87-91.

Benedict CR, Johnstone DE, Weiner DH, Bourassa MG, Bittner V, Kay R, Kirlin P, Greenberg B, Kohn RM, Mickias JM, McIntyre K, Quinones MA, Yusuf S. 1994. Relation of neurohumoral activation to clinical variables and degree of ventricular dysfunction: A report from the registry of studies of left ventricular dysfunction. *J Am Coll Cardiol* 23:1410-1420.

Bersin RM, Kwasman M, Lau D, Klinski C, Tanaka K, Khorrami P, DeMarco T, Wolfe C, Chatterjee K. 1993. Importance of oxygen-haemoglobin binding to oxygen transport in congestive heart failure. *Br Heart J* 70:443-447.

Bertolet BD, Pepine CJ. 1995. Daily life cardiac ischemia: Should it be treated? *Drugs* 49:176-195.

Blankenhorn DH, Nessim SA, Johnson RL, Sanmarco ME, Azon SP, Cashin-Hemphill L. 1987. Beneficial effects of combined colestipol-niacin therapy on coronary atherosclerosis and coronary venous bypass grafts. *JAMA* 257:3233-3240.

Brady JA, Rock CL, Horneffer MR. 1995. Thiamin status, diuretic medications, and the management of congestive heart failure. *J Am Diet Assoc* 95:541-544.

Braunwald E, Sobel BE. 1988. Coronary blood flow and myocardial ischemia. In *Textbook of Cardiovascular Medicine*. 3rd ed. Braunwald E (ed). Philadelphia: W.B. Saunders, pp.1191-1221.

Bristow MR, Gilbert EM, Abraham WT, Adams KF, Fowler MB, Hershberger RE, Kubo SH, Narahara KA, Ingersoll H, Krueger S, Young S, Shusterman N. 1996. Carvedilol produces dose-related improvements in left ventricular function and survival in subjects with chronic heart failure. *Circulation* 94:2807-2816.

Bristow MR, O'Connel JB, Gilbert EM, French WJ, Leatherman G, Kantrowitz NE, Orie J, Smucker ML, Marshall G, Kelly P, Deitchman D, Anderson JL. 1994. Dose-response of chronic beta blocker treatment in heart failure from either idiopathic dilated or ischemic cardiomyopathy. *Circulation* 89:1632-1642.

Buchwald H, Matts JP, Fitch LL, Campos CT, Sanmarco ME, Amplatz K, Castaneda-Zuniga WR, Hunter DW, Pearce MB, Bissett JK, Edmiston WA, Savin HS Jr, Weber FJ, Varco RL, Campbell GS, Yellin AE, Smink RD Jr, Long JM, Hansen BJ, Chalmers TC, Meier P, Stamler J. For the program on the surgical control of the hyperlipidemias (POSCH) group. 1992. Changes in sequential coronary arteriograms and subsequent coronary events. *JAMA* 268:1429-1437.

Cardiology Preeminence Roundtable. 1994. *Beyond Four Walls: Cost-Effective Management of Chronic Congestive Heart Failure.* Washington, D.C.: Advisory Board Company.

Chesebro JH, Zoldhelyi P, Fuster V. 1991. Plaque disruption and thrombosis in unstable angina pectoris. *Am J Cardiol* 68:9C-15C.

Cleland JGF. 1994. The clinical course of heart failure and its modification by ACE inhibitors: Insights from recent clinical trials. *Eur Heart J* 15:125-130.

Codd MB, Sugrue DD, Gersh BJ, Melton LJ. 1989. Epidemiology of dilated and hypertrophic cardiomyopathy: A population-based study in Olmsted County, Minnesota, 1975-1984. *Circulation* 80:564-572.

Cohn JN. 1995. Structural basis for heart failure: Ventricular remodeling and its pharmacologic inhibition. *Circulation* 91:2504-2507.

Cohn JN, Bristow MR, Chien KR, Colucci WS, Frazier OH, Leinwand LA, Lorell BH, Moss AJ, Sonnenblick EH, Walsh RA, Mockrin SC, Reinlib L. 1997. Report of the National Heart, Lung and Blood Institute special emphasis panel on heart failure research. *Circulation* 95:766-770.

Colucci WS, Packer M, Bristow MR, Gilbert EM, Cohn JN, Fowler MB, Krueger SK, Hershberger R, Uretsky BF, Bowers JA, Sackner-Bernstein JD, Young ST, Holeslaw TL, Lukas MA. 1996. Carvedilol inhibits clinical progression in patients with mild symptoms of heart failure. *Circulation* 94:2800-2806.

de Divitiis M, Rubba P, DiSomma S, Liguori V, Galderisi M, Montefusco S, Carreras G, Greco V, Carotenuto A, Iannuzzo G, de Divitiis O. 1996. Effects of short-term reduction in serum cholesterol with simvastatin in patients with stable angina pectoris and mild to moderate hypercholesterolemia. *Am J Cardiol* 78:763-768.

de Lorgeril M, Salen P, Martin JL, Mamelle N, Monjaud I, Touboul P, Delaye J. 1996. Effect of a Mediterranean type of diet on the rate of cardiovascular complications in patients with coronary artery disease: Insights into the cardioprotective effect of certain nutrients. *J Am Coll Cardiol* 28:1103-1108.

Demopoulos L, LeJemtel TH. 1994. Peripheral factors in the management of congestive heart failure. *Cardiovascular Drugs and Therapy* 8:75-82.

Dickstein K, Chang P, Willenheimer R, Haunso S, Remes J, Hall C, Kjekshus J. 1995. Comparison of the effects of losartin and enalapril on clinical status and exercise performance in patients with moderate or severe chronic heart failure. *J Am Coll Cardiol* 26:438-445.

Dracup K, Baker DW, Dunbar SB, Dacey RA, Brooks NH, Johnson JC, Oken C, Massie BM. 1994. Management of heart failure II: Counseling, education, and lifestyle modifications. *JAMA* 272:1442-1446.

Dries DL, Domanski MJ, Waclawiw MA, Gersh BJ. 1997. Effect of antithrombotic therapy on risk of sudden coronary death in patients with congestive heart failure. *Am J Cardiol* 79:909-913.

Duncan AK, Vittone J, Fleming KC, Smith HC. 1996. Cardiovascular disease in elderly patients. *Mayo Clin Proc* 71:184-196.

Egashira K, Hirooka Y, Kai H, Sugimachi M, Suzuki S, Inou A, Takeshita A. 1994. Reduction in serum cholesterol with pravastatin improves endo-thelium-dependent coronary vasomotion in patients with hypercholester-olemia. *Circulation* 89:2519-2524.

Eichhorn EJ, Bristow MR. 1996. Medical therapy can improve the biological properties of the chronically failing heart: A new era in the treatment of heart failure. *Circulation* 94:2285-2296.

Enriquez-Sarano M, Rossi A, Seward JB, Bailey KR, Tajik AJ. 1997. Determinants of pulmonary hypertension in left ventricular dysfunction. *J Am Coll Cardiol* 29:153-159.

Erlemeier HH, Kupper W, Bleifeld W. 1992. Intermittent infusion of dobutamine in the therapy of severe congestive heart failure: Long-term effects and lack of tolerance. *Cardiovascular Drugs and Therapy* 6:391-398.

Evans SA, Watson L, Hawkins M, Cowley AJ, Johnston IDA, Kinnear WJM. 1995. Respiratory muscle strength in chronic heart failure. *Thorax* 50:625-628.

Expert Panel on Detection, Evaluation, and Treatment of High Blood Cholesterol in Adults. 1993. Summary of the second report of the National Cholesterol Education Program (NCEP) expert panel on detection, evalua-tion, and treatment of high blood cholesterol in adults (Adult Treatment Panel II). *JAMA* 269:3015-3023.

Falk E, Shah PK, Fuster V. 1995. Coronary plaque disruption. *Circulation* 92:657-671.

Ferrari R. 1995. Metabolic disturbances during myocardial ischemia and reperfusion. *Am J Cardiol* 76:17B-24B.

Ferrari R, Bachetti T, Confortini R, Opasich C, Febo O, Corti A, Cassani G, Visioli O. 1995. Tumor necrosis factor soluble receptors in patients with various degrees of congestive heart failure. *Circulation* 92:1479-1486.

Francis GS, McDonald K, Chu C, Cohn JN. 1995. Pathophysiologic aspects of end-stage heart failure. *Am J Cardiol* 75:11A-16A.

Franklin BA. 1991. Exercise training and coronary collateral circulation. *Med Sci Sports Exerc* 23:648-653.

Friedman M, Breall WS, Goodwin ML, Sparagen BJ, Ghandour G, Fleischmann N. 1996. Effect of type A behavioral counseling on frequency of episodes of silent myocardial ischemia in coronary patients. *Am Heart J* 132:933-937.

Gaasch WH. 1994. Diagnosis and treatment of heart failure based on left ventricular systolic or diastolic dysfunction *JAMA* 271:1276-1280.

Gagliardi JA, Prado NG, Marino JC, Lederer S, Ramos AO, Bertolasi CA. 1996. Exercise training and heparin pretreatment in patients with coronary artery disease. *Am Heart J* 132:946-951.

Garg R, Yusuf S. 1995. Overview of randomized trials of angiotensin-converting enzyme inhibitors on mortality and morbidity in patients with heart failure. *JAMA* 273:1450-1456.

Garratt KN, Morgan JP. 1991. Coronary circulation: B. Pathophysiology of myocardial ischemia and reperfusion. In *Cardiology: Fundamentals and Practice*. Giuliani ER, Fuster V, Gersh BJ, McGoon MD, McGoon DC (eds). St. Louis: Mosby, pp. 1150-1158.

Garratt KN, Reeder GS, Holmes DR. 1996. Cardiac catheterization and angiography: B. Interventional cardiac therapy. In *Mayo Clinic Practice of Cardiology*. 3rd ed. Giuliani ER, Gersh BJ, McGoon MD, Hayes DL, Schaff HV (eds). St. Louis: Mosby, pp. 366-399.

Gerhard M, Ganz P. 1995. How do we explain the clinical benefits of estrogen? from bedside to bench. *Circulation* 92:5-8.

Goldman, L, Hashimoto B, Cook EF, Loscalzo A. 1981. Comparative reproducibility and validity of systems for assessing cardiovascular functional class: Advantages of a new specific activity scale. *Circulation* 64:1227-1234.

Goode GF, Heagerty AM. 1995. In vitro responses of human peripheral small arteries in hypercholesterolemia and effects of therapy. *Circulation* 91:2898-2903.

Gotto AM. 1995. Lipid lowering, regression, and coronary events: A review of the interdisciplinary council on lipids and cardiovascular risk intervention. Seventh council meeting. *Circulation* 92:646-656.

Gould KL. 1994. Reversal of coronary atherosclerosis: Clinical promise as the basis for noninvasive management of coronary artery disease. *Circulation* 90:1558-1571.

Gould KL, Ornish D, Scherwitz L, Brown S, Edens RP, Hess MJ, Mullani N, Bolomey L, Dobbs F, Armstrong WT, Merritt T, Ports T, Sparler S, Billings J. 1995. Changes in myocardial perfusion abnormalities by positron emission tomography after long-term, intense risk factor modification. *JAMA* 274:894-901.

Grady KL, Jalowiec A, Grusk BB, White-Williams C, Robinson JA. 1992. Symptom distress in cardiac transplant candidates. *Heart Lung* 21:434-439.

Grassi G, Servalle G, Cattaneo BM, Lanfranchi A, Vailati S, Giannattasio C, Del Bo A, Sala C, Bolla GB, Pozzi M, Mancia G. 1995. Sympathetic activation and loss of reflex sympathetic control in mild congestive heart failure. *Circulation* 92:3206-3211.

Greenberg B, Quinones MA, Koilpillai C, Limacher M, Shindler D, Benedict C, Shelton B. 1995. Effects of long-term enalapril therapy on cardiac structure and function in patients with left ventricular dysfunction: Results of the SOLVD echocardiography substudy. *Circulation* 91:2573-2581.

Grimm M, Yeganehfar W, Laufer G, Madl C, Kramer L, Eisenhuber E, Simon P, Kupilik N, Schreiner W, Pacher R, Bunzel B, Wolner E, Grimm G. 1996. Cyclosporine may affect improvement of cognitive brain function after successful cardiac transplantation. *Circulation* 94:1339-1345.

Grodstein F, Stampfer MJ, Manson JE, Colditz GA, Willett WC, Rosner B, Speizer FE, Hennekens CH. 1996. Postmenopausal estrogen and progestin use and the risk of cardiovascular disease. *N Eng J Med* 335:453-461.

Guetta V, Cannon RO. 1996. Cardiovascular effects of estrogen and lipid-lowering therapies in postmenopausal women. *Circulation* 93:1928-1937.

Guyton AC. 1986. *Textbook of Medical Physiology.* 7th ed. Philadelphia: WB Saunders, pp. 296-298.

Hambrecht R, Niebauer J, Marburger C, Grunze M, Kalberer B, Hauer K, Schlierf G, Kubler W, Schuler G. 1993. Various intensities of leisure time physical activity in patients with coronary artery disease: Effects on cardio-respiratory fitness and progression of coronary atherosclerotic lesions. *J Am Coll Cardiol* 22:468-477.

Henry PD, Cabello OA, Chew CH. 1995. Hypercholesterolemia and endothelial dysfunction. *Current Opinion in Lipidology* 6:190-195.

Herrlin B, Sylven C. 1991. Increased arterial oxygen content: An important compensatory mechanism in chronic heart failure. *Cardiovascular Research* 25:384-390.

Hurst JW. 1992. Coronary heart disease: The overview of the clinician. In *Rehabilitation of the Coronary Patient.* 3rd ed. Wenger NK, Hellerstein HK (eds). New York: Churchill Livingston, pp. 3-18.

Kannel WB, Belanger AJ. 1991. Epidemiology of heart failure. *Am Heart J* 121:951-957.

Karon BL. 1995. Diagnosis and outpatient management of congestive heart failure. *Mayo Clin Proc* 70:1080-1085.

Katz AM. 1993. Metabolism of the failing heart. *Cardioscience* 4:199-203.

Kaye DM, Lefkovitz J, Jennings GL, Bergin P, Broughton A, Esler MD. 1995. Adverse consequences of high sympathetic nervous activity in the failing human heart. *J Am Coll Cardiol* 26:1257-1263.

Kottke TE, Weidman WH, Nguyen TT. 1996. Prevention of coronary heart disease. In *Mayo Clinic Practice of Cardiology.* 3rd ed. Giuliani ER, Gersh BJ, McGoon MD, Hayes DL, Schaff HV (eds). St. Louis: Mosby, pp. 490-528.

Krum H, Goldsmith R, Wilshire-Clement M, Miller M, Packer M. 1995a. Role of endothelin in the exercise intolerance of chronic heart failure. *Am J Cardiol* 75:1282-1283.

Krum H, Sackner-Bernstein JD, Goldsmith RL, Kukin ML, Schwartz B, Penn J, Medina N, Yushak M, Horn E, Katz SD, Levin HR, Neuberg GW, Delong G, Packer M. 1995b. Double-blind, placebo-controlled study of the long-term efficacy of carvedilol in patients with severe chronic heart failure. *Circulation* 92:1499-1506.

Laslett LJ, Paumer L, Amsterdam EA. 1985. Increase in myocardial oxygen consumption index by exercise training at the onset of ischemia in patients with coronary artery disease. *Circulation* 71:958-962.

Leor J, Kloner RA. 1995. The Northridge earthquake as a trigger for acute myocardial infarction. *Am J Cardiol* 77:1230-1232.

Leor J, Pool WK, Kloner RA. 1996. Sudden cardiac death triggered by an earthquake. *N Eng J Med* 334:413-419.

Levine GN, Frei B, Koulouris SN, Gerhard MD, Keaney JF, Vita JA. 1996. Ascorbic acid reverses endothelial vasomotor dysfunction in patients with coronary artery disease. *Circulation* 93:1107-1113.

Lie JJ. 1991. Atherosclerosis B. Pathology of coronary artery disease. In *Cardiology, Fundamentals and Practice*. 2nd ed. Giuliani ER, Fuster V, Gersh BJ, McGoon MD, McGoon DC (eds). Chicago: Mosby, pp. 1211-1231.

Linden W, Stossel C, Maurice J. 1996. Psychosocial interventions for patients with coronary artery disease: A meta-analysis. *Arch Intern Med* 156:745-752.

Lommi J, Kupari M, Koskinen P, Naveri H, Leinonen H, Pulkki K, Harkonen M. 1996. Blood ketone bodies in congestive heart failure. *J Am Coll Cardiol* 28:665-672.

Magovern JA, Magovern GJ, Maher TD, Benckart DH, Park SB, Christlieb LY, Magovern GJ Jr. 1993. Operation for congestive heart failure: Transplantation, coronary artery bypass, and cardiomyoplasty. *Ann Thorac Surg* 56:418-425.

Mancini DM, Davis L, Wexler JP, Chadwick B, LeJemtel TH. 1987. Dependence of enhanced maximal exercise performance on increased peak skeletal muscle perfusion during long-term captopril therapy in heart failure. *J Am Coll Cardiol* 10:845-850.

Mancini DM, Henson D, LaManca J, Levine S. 1994. Evidence of reduced respiratory muscle endurance in patients with heart failure. *J Am Coll Cardiol* 24:972-981.

Mancini GBJ, Henry GC, Macaya C, O'Neill BJ, Pucillo AL, Carere RG, Wargovich TJ, Mudra H, Luscher TF, Klibaner MI, Haber HE, Uprichard ACG, Pepine CJ, Pitt B. 1996. Angiotensin-converting enzyme inhibition with quinipril improves endothelial vasomotor function in patients with coronary artery disease: The TREND (trial on reversing endothelial dysfunction) study. *Circulation* 94:258-265.

Massie BM. 1994. A personal perspective on the treatment of heart failure in 1994. *Current Opinion in Cardiology* 9:225-263.

Massie BM, Simonini A, Sahgal P, Wells L, Dudley GA. 1996. Relation of systemic and local muscle exercise capacity to skeletal muscle characteristics in men with congestive heart failure. *J Am Coll Cardiol* 27:140-145.

McGoon MD, Fuster V, Gersh BJ, Mullany CJ. 1996. Coronary revascularization: Indications and outcomes. In *Mayo Clinic Practice of Cardiology*. 3rd ed. Giuliani ER, Gersh BJ, McGoon MD, Hayes DL, Schaff HV (eds). St. Louis: Mosby, pp. 1387-1397.

McGoon MD, Shub C. 1996. Myocardial ischemia clinical syndromes. C. Antianginal agents. In *Mayo Clinic Practice of Cardiology*. 3rd ed. Giuliani ER, Gersh BJ, McGoon MD, Hayes DL, Schaff HV (eds). St. Louis: Mosby, pp. 1191-1213.

Moreira LFP, Seferian P, Bocchi EA, Pego-Fernandez PM, Stolf NAG, Pereira-Barretto AC, Jatene AD. 1991. Survival improvement with dynamic cardiomyoplasty in patients with dilated cardiomyopathy. *Circulation* 84(Suppl III):296-302.

Moruzzi P, Doria E, Agostoni PG. 1996. Medium term effectiveness of L-thyroxine treatment in idiopathic dilated cardiomyopathy. *Am J Med* 101:461-467.

Moss AJ, Hall WJ, Cannom DS, Daubert JP, Higgins SL, Klein H, Levine JH, Saksena S, Waldo AL, Wilber D, Brown MW, Heo M. 1996. Improved survival with an implanted defibrillator in patients with coronary disease at high risk for ventricular arrhythmia. *N Eng J Med* 335:1933-1940.

Niebauer J, Hambrecht R, Marburger C, Hauer K, Velich T, von Hodenberg E, Schlierf G, Kubler W, Schuler G. 1995. Impact of intensive physical exercise and low-fat diet on collateral vessel formation in stable angina pectoris and angiographically confirmed coronary artery disease. *Am J Cardiol* 76:771-775.

Nishimoto Y, Firth BR, Kloner RA, Loer J, Lerman RD, Bhandari AK, Cannom DS. 1995. The 1994 Northridge earthquake triggered shocks from implantable cardioverter defibrillators. *Circulation* 92(Suppl I Abstract): 605-606.

Nishimura RA, Symanski JD, Hurrell DG, Trusty JM, Hayes DL, Tajik AJ. 1996. Dual-chamber pacing for cardiomyopathies: A 1996 clinical perspective. *Mayo Clin Proc* 71:1077-1087.

Oka RK, Stotts NA, Dae MW, Haskell WL, Gortner SR. 1993. Daily physical activity levels in congestive heart failure. *Am J Cardiol* 71:921-925.

Olson LJ, Miller WL. 1996. Pharmacotherapy of congestive heart failure. In *Mayo Clinic Practice of Cardiology*. 3rd ed. Giuliani ER, Gersh BJ, McGoon MD, Hayes DL, Schaff HV (eds). St. Louis: Mosby, pp. 588-622.

Opie LH. 1995. Fundamental role of angiotensin-converting enzyme inhibitors in the management of congestive heart failure. *Am J Cardiol* 75:3F-6F.

Ornish D, Brown SE, Scherwitz LW, Billings JH, Armstrong WT, Ports TA, McLanahaw SM, Kirkeeide RL, Brand RJ, Gould KL. 1990. Can lifestyle changes reverse coronary heart disease? the lifestyle heart trial. *Lancet* 336:129-133.

Packer M. 1990. Abnormalities of diastolic function as a potential cause of exercise intolerance in chronic heart failure. *Circulation* 81(Suppl III):78-86.

Packer M. 1995. Is tumor necrosis factor an important neurohormonal mechanism in chronic heart failure? *Circulation* 92:1379-1382.

Packer M, Bristow MR, Cohn JN, Colucci WS, Fowler MB, Gilbert EM, Shusterman NH. 1996a. The effect of carvedilol on morbidity and mortality in patients with chronic heart failure. *N Eng J Med* 334:1349-1355.

Packer M, Colucci WS, Sackner-Bernstein JD, Liang CS, Goldscher DA, Freeman I, Kukin ML, Kinhal V, Udelson JE, Klapholz M, Gottlieb SS, Pearle D, Cody RJ, Gregory JJ, Kantrowitz NE, LeJemtel TH, Young ST, Lukas MA, Shusterman NH. 1996b. Double-blind, placebo-controlled study of the effects of carvedilol in patients with moderate to severe heart failure: The PRECISE trial. *Circulation* 94:2793-2799.

Pitt B. 1997. The potential use of angiotensin-converting enzyme inhibitors in patients with hyperlipidemia. *Am J Cardiol* 79(5A):24-28.

Raffo JA, Luksic IY, Kappagoda CT, Mary DASG, Whitaker W, Linden RJ. 1980. Effects of physical training on myocardial ischemia in patients with coronary artery disease. *Br Heart J* 43:262-269.

Rahimtoola SH. 1995. From coronary artery disease to heart failure: Role of the hibernating myocardium. *Am J Cardiol* 75:16E-22E.

Raman VK, Lee YA, Lindpainter K. 1995. The cardiac renin-angiotensin-aldosterone system and hypertensive cardiac hypertrophy. *Am J Cardiol* 76:18D-23D.

Rector TS, Bank AJ, Mullen KA, Tschumperlin LK, Sih R, Pillai K, Kubo SH. 1996. Randomized, double-blind, placebo-controlled study of supplemental oral L-arginine in patients with heart failure. *Circulation* 93:2135-2141.

Redfield MM. 1996. Evaluation of congestive heart failure. In *Mayo Clinic Practice of Cardiology*. 3rd ed. Giuliani ER, Gersh BJ, McGoon MD, Hayes DL, Schaff HV (eds). St. Louis: Mosby, pp. 569-587.

Redfield MM, Gersh BJ, Bailey KR, Rodeheffer RJ. 1994. Natural history of incidentally discovered, asymptomatic idiopathic dilated cardiomyopathy. *Am J Cardiol* 74:737-739.

Rich MW, Beckham R, Wittenberg C, Leven CL, Freedland KE, Carney RM. 1995. A multidisciplinary intervention to prevent the readmission of elderly patients with congestive heart failure. *N Eng J Med* 333:1190-1195.

Rodeheffer RJ, Gersh BJ. 1996. Cardiomyopathy and biopsy. A. Dilated cardiomyopathy and the myocarditides. In *Mayo Clinic Practice of Cardiology*. 3rd ed. Giuliani ER, Gersh BJ, McGoon MD, Hayes DL, Schaff HV (eds). St. Louis: Mosby, pp. 636-671.

Rodeheffer RJ, Miller WL, Burnett JC. 1996. Pathophysiology of circulatory failure. In *Mayo Clinic Practice of Cardiology*. 3rd ed. Giuliani ER, Gersh BJ, McGoon MD, Hayes DL, Schaff HV (eds). St. Louis: Mosby, pp. 550-568.

Rogers WJ, Johnstone DE, Yusuf S, Weiner DH, Gallagher P, Bittner VA, Ahn S, Schrow E, Shumaker SA, Sheffield LT. 1994. Quality of life among 5,025 patients with left ventricular dysfunction randomized between placebo and enalapril: The studies of left ventricular dysfunction. *J Am Coll Cardiol* 23:393-400.

Ross R. 1988. The pathogenesis of atherosclerosis. In *Heart Disease: A Textbook of Cardiovascular Medicine*. 3rd ed. Braunwald E (ed). Philadelphia: WB Saunders, pp. 1135-1152.

Rossouw JE. 1996. Estrogens for prevention of coronary heart disease: Putting the brakes on the bandwagon. *Circulation* 94:2982-2985.

Scandinavian Simvastatin Survival Study Group. 1994. Randomized trial of cholesterol lowering in 4,444 patients with coronary heart disease: The Scandinavian simvastatin survival study (4S). *Lancet* 344:1383-1389.

Schuler G, Schlierf G, Wirth A, Mautner HP, Scheurlen H, Thumm M, Roth H, Scharz F, Kohlmeier M, Mehmel HC, Kubler W. 1988. Low-fat diet and regular, supervised physical exercise in patients with symptomatic coronary artery disease: Reduction of stress-induced myocardial ischemia. *Circulation* 77:172-181.

Seiler C, Suter TM, Hess OM. 1995. Exercise-induced vasomotion of angiographically normal and stenotic coronary arteries improves after cholesterol-lowering drug therapy with bezafibrate. *J Am Coll Cardiol* 26:1615-1622.

Senni M, Redfield MM. 1997. Congestive heart failure in elderly patients. *Mayo Clinic Proc* 72:453-460.

Shimon I, Almog S, Vered Z, Seligmann H, Shefi M, Peleg E, Rosenthal T, Motro M, Halkin H, Ezra D. 1995. Improved left ventricular function after thiamin supplementation in patients with congestive heart failure receiving long-term furosemide therapy. *Am J Med* 98:485-490.

Shub C. 1991. Myocardial ischemia syndromes. A. Heart disease. In *Cardiology: Fundamentals and Practice*. Giuliani ER, Fuster V, Gersh BJ, McGoon MD, McGoon DC (eds). St. Louis: Mosby, pp. 1276-1306.

Soler-Soler J, Permanyer-Miralda G. 1994. How do changes in lifestyle complement medical treatment in heart failure? *Br Heart J* 72(suppl):87-91.

Squires RW. 1995. Mechanisms by which exercise training may improve the clinical status of cardiac patients. In *Heart Disease and Rehabilitation*. 3rd ed. Pollock ML, Schmidt DH (eds). Champaign, IL: Human Kinetics, pp. 147-160.

Squires RW, Gau GT, Miller TD, Allison TG, Morris PB. 1996. Cardiac rehabilitation and cardiovascular health enhancement. In *Mayo Clinic Practice of Cardiology*. 3rd ed. Giuliani ER, Gersh BJ, McGoon MD, Hayes DL, Schaff HV (eds). St. Louis: Mosby, pp. 529-549.

Squires RW, Williams WL. 1993. Coronary atherosclerosis and myocardial infarction. In *The American College of Sports Medicine. ACSM's Resource Manual for Guidelines for Exercise Testing and Prescription*. 2nd ed. Philadelphia: Lea & Febiger, pp. 168-186.

Stark RM. 1996. Review of the major intervention trials of lowering coronary artery disease risk through cholesterol reduction. *Am J Cardiol* 78(Suppl 6A):13-19.

Stephens NG, Parsons A, Schofield PM, Cheeseman K, Mitchinson MJ, Brown MJ. 1996. Randomized controlled trial of vitamin E in patients with coronary disease: Cambridge heart antioxidant study (CHAOS). *Lancet* 347:781-786.

Stevenson JC, Crook D, Godsland IF, Collins P, Whitcherd MI. 1994. Hormone replacement therapy and the cardiovascular system: Nonlipid effects. *Drugs* 47(suppl 2):35-41.

Sullivan M, Atwood JE, Myers J, Feuer J, Hall P, Kellerman B, Forbes S, Froelicher V. 1989. Increased exercise capacity after digoxin administration in patients with heart failure. *J Am Coll Cardiol* 13:1138-1143.

The Pimobendan in Congestive Heart Failure (PICO) Investigators. 1996. Effect of pimobendan on exercise capacity in patients with chronic heart failure: Main results from the pimobendan in congestive heart failure (PICO) trial. *Heart* 76:223-231.

Todd IC, Brandnam MS, Cooke MBD, Ballantyne D. 1991. Effects of daily high-intensity exercise on myocardial perfusion in angina pectoris. *Am J Cardiol* 68:1593-1599.

Topol EJ, Nissen SE. 1995. Our preoccupation with coronary lumenology: The dissociation between clinical and angiographic findings in ischemic heart disease. *Circulation* 92:2333-2342.

Torre-Amione G, Kapadia S, Benedict C, Oral H, Young JB, Mann DL. 1996a. Proinflammatory cytokine levels in patients with depressed left ventricular ejection fraction: A report from the studies of left ventricular dysfunction (SOLVD). *J Am Coll Cardiol* 27:1201-1206.

Torre-Amione G, Kapadia S, Lee J, Durand JB, Bies RD, Young JB, Mann DL. 1996b. Tumor necrosis factor-alpha and tumor necrosis factor receptors in the failing human heart. *Circulation* 93:704-711.

Trappe SW, Costill DL, Fink WJ, Pearson DR. 1995. Skeletal muscle characteristics among distance runners: A 20 yr follow-up study. *J Appl Physiol* 78:823-829.

Treasure CB, Klein JL, Weintraub WS, Talley JD, Stillabower ME, Kosinski AS, Zhang J, Boccuzzi SJ, Cedarholm JC, Alexander RW. 1995. Beneficial effects of cholesterol-lowering therapy on the coronary endothelium in patients with coronary artery disease. *N Eng J Med*. 332:481-487.

Vasan RS, Benjamin EJ, Levy D. 1995. Prevalence, clinical features, and prognosis of diastolic heart failure: An epidemiologic perspective. *J Am Coll Cardiol* 26:1565-1574.

Waters D, Higginson L, Gladstone P, Boccuzzi SJ, Cook T, Lesperance J. 1995. Effects of cholesterol lowering on the progression of coronary atherosclerosis in women: A Canadian coronary atherosclerosis intervention trial (CCAIT) substudy. *Circulation* 92:2404-2410.

Wei CM, Lerman A, Rodeheffer RJ, McGregor CGA, Brandt RR, Wright S, Heublein DM, Kao PC, Edwards WD, Brunett JC. 1994. Endothelin in human congestive heart failure. *Circulation* 89:1580-1586.

Zamarra JW, Schneider RH, Besseghini I, Robinson DK, Salerno JW. 1996. Usefulness of the Transcendental Meditation program in the treatment of patients with coronary artery disease. *Am J Cardiol* 77:867-870.

Zeiher AM, Krause T, Schachinger V, Minners J, Moser E. 1995. Impaired endothelium-dependent vasodilation of coronary resistance vessels in association with exercise-induced myocardial ischemia. *Circulation* 91:2345-2352.

CHAPTER 3

Acute Exercise and Exercise Testing in Myocardial Ischemia and Chronic Heart Failure

This chapter reviews the abnormal responses of the cardiovascular system to an acute bout of exercise in patients who have coronary artery disease with exercise-related ischemia or with left ventricular dysfunction. It also discusses graded exercise testing techniques. Examples of data from various types of exercise tests are presented with the case studies in chapter 5.

Acute Exercise Responses in Myocardial Ischemia

Myocardial ischemia, depending upon the severity and the amount of cardiac muscle involved, may cause derangement of the oxygen transport system and impairment of exercise capacity. However, not all patients with myocardial ischemia will have compromised oxygen transport. The following abnormal exercise responses may be observed in patients with ischemia.

Coronary Vasoconstriction

In patients with coronary artery disease, an acute bout of exercise may cause constriction of diseased coronary arterial segments, increasing the likelihood of exercise-related myocardial ischemia. The mechanism responsible for this vasoconstriction is not completely understood but it may be related to elevated plasma catecholamine concentrations, a subnormal production of endothelium-derived vasorelaxing factor (nitric oxide), or platelet aggregation with release of thromboxane A2, a potent vasoconstrictor (Hess et al. 1990). Exercise may increase levels of endothelin, a powerful vasoconstrictor, in patients with coronary atherosclerosis, but not in persons with healthy coronary arteries (Predel et al. 1995).

Ventricular Systolic and Diastolic Dysfunction

Ischemia may reduce the effectiveness of ventricular pump function (Squires and Williams 1993; Hurst 1992). Left and right ventricular ejection fractions may decrease during exercise (normal response is an increase in ejection fraction), regional wall-motion abnormalities may develop in ischemic portions of the myocardium, diastolic filling may be impaired as a result of a reduction in compliance of the ventricles (increased stiffness), and stroke volume may not increase normally during exercise. Figure 3.1 compares left ventricular ejection fraction and peak ventricular emptying rate for normal subjects and patients with substantial exercise-induced ischemia.

Note both the decrease in ejection fraction and emptying rate for patients with ischemia and the rather prompt recovery of global systolic function at the conclusion of exercise. Regional wall motion, which worsens with acute exercise, may require one to two hours to return to pre-exercise levels (Ambrosio et al. 1996). However, as shown in figure 3.2, diastolic function, as measured by the ventricular filling rate, is depressed not only during exercise under severely ischemic conditions but potentially for several days.

Oxygen Transport System

Hossack (1987) compared the oxygen transport systems (Fick equation) of normal controls and patients with coronary artery disease during treadmill exercise with hemodynamic (arterial and right atrial catheters) and cardiopulmonary measurements (see figure 3.3).

The greatest difference between patients and controls was for aerobic capacity, with a mean $\dot{V}O_2$max of 48% of normal for the patients. Maximal cardiac output was 57% of normal. Both heart rate and stroke volume were lower, on average, for patients than controls. The blunted heart rate response to exercise observed in some patients with ischemia is independent of medication effects. In fact, in some patients with right coronary artery disease and exercise-related ischemia, heart rate may actually decrease (sinus node deceleration) at some point during graded exercise testing (Miller et al. 1993). Arterial-mixed venous oxygen difference was also lower for the patients, in the study of Hossack.

It should be emphasized that the magnitude of the impairment in oxygen transport is highly variable. For patients with a history of myocardial infarction, infarct size does correlate positively with exercise capacity (Carter and Amundsen 1977). Patients with myocardial ischemia usually have slower $\dot{V}O_2$ kinetics with a lower $\dot{V}O_2$ at any point during an incremental exercise test compared with normal individuals. This

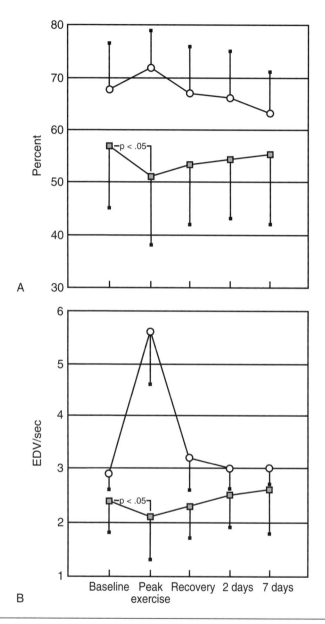

Figure 3.1 Left ventricular ejection fraction (A) and peak ventricular empty-ing rate (B) at baseline, at peak exercise, during immediate recovery from peak exercise, and at 2 and 7 days postexercise in control subjects (○) and patients with ischemic heart disease (■). EDV = end-diastolic volume.

Reprinted from *Journal of the American College of Cardiology*, 17, Fragasso G, Benti R, Sciammarella M, Rossetti E, Savi A, Gerundini P, Chierchia SL., Symptom-limited exercise testing causes sustained diastolic dysfunction in patients with coronary disease and low effort tolerance, 1254, Copyright 1991, with permission from the American College of Cardiology.

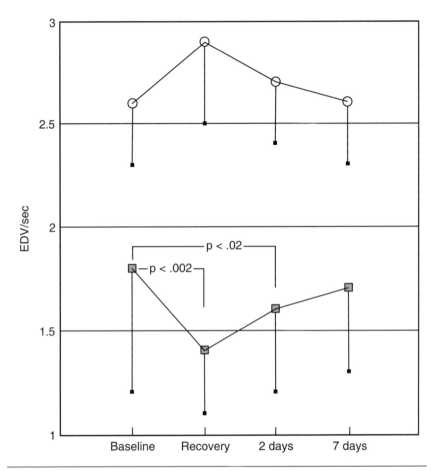

Figure 3.2   Left ventricular filling rate at baseline, during immediate recovery from peak exercise, and at 2 and 7 days postexercise in control subjects (○) and in patients with ischemic heart disease (■). EDV = end-diastolic volume.

Reprinted from *Journal of the American College of Cardiology*, 17, Fragasso G, Benti R, Sciammarella M, Rossetti E, Savi A, Gerundini P, Chierchia SL., Symptom-limited exercise testing causes sustained diastolic dysfunction in patients with coronary disease and low effort tolerance, 1254, Copyright 1991, with permission from the American College of Cardiology.

makes estimating $\dot{V}O_2$ from treadmill time or workload problematic. The patients with slower $\dot{V}O_2$ kinetics have a greater reliance on anaerobic energy production during exercise. Treatment of ischemia with medications such as calcium channel antagonists improves oxygen uptake kinetics, as demonstrated in figure 3.4.

Systolic and Diastolic Blood Pressure

Most patients with coronary artery disease and exercise-induced myocardial ischemia exhibit a normal blood pressure response to aerobic exercise.

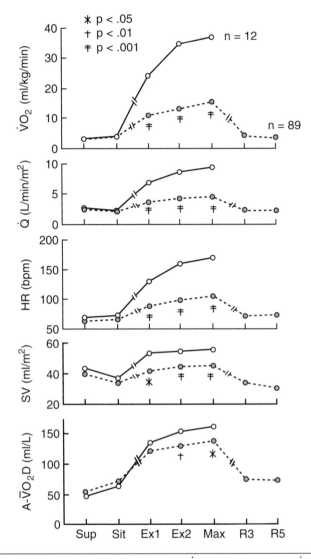

Figure 3.3   Mean values for oxygen uptake ($\dot{V}O_2$), cardiac index ($\dot{Q}$), heart rate (HR), stroke volume (SV), and arterial-mixed venous oxygen difference (A-$\overline{V}O_2D$) for control subjects (○) and patients with coronary artery disease (●).
Reprinted, with permission, from Hossack KF. Cardiovascular responses to dynamic exercise. 1987. *Cardiology Clinics* 5:147-156. Copyright 1987 W.B. Saunders Company.

However, some patients demonstrate either hypotensive or hypertensive responses. The most serious abnormal blood pressure response is systolic hypotension with an exercise blood pressure lower than the pre-exercise pressure (Iskandrian et al. 1992). Patients with a hypotensive systolic blood pressure response to graded exercise are at higher risk for a cardiac event.

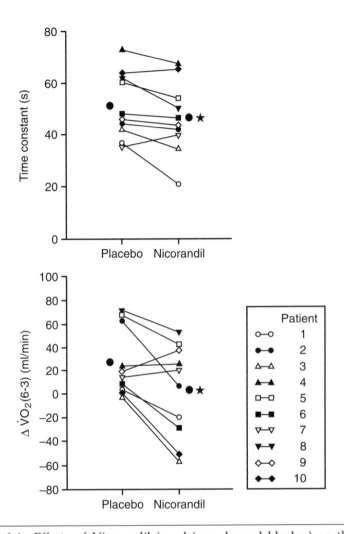

Figure 3.4   Effects of Nicorandil (a calcium channel blocker) on the time constant for oxygen uptake ($\dot{V}O_2$), and the increase in $\dot{V}O_2$ at six minutes compared with three minutes during constant intensity exercise. ★ $p < .05$.

Reprinted from *The American Journal of Cardiology*, 76, Koike A, Hiroe M, Yajima T, Adachi H, Shimizu N, Kano H, Sugimoto K, Miyahara Y, Korenaga M, Marumo F., Effects of Nicorandil on kinetics of oxygen uptake at the onset of exercise in patients with coronary artery disease, 451, Copyright 1995, with permission from Excerpta Medica Inc.

The mechanisms responsible for the hypotensive response are speculative. However, cardiac output seldom decreases during exercise, even in patients with severe ischemia. Neurogenic reflex vasodilation involving mechanoreceptors in the myocardium (Bezold-Jarisch reflex) may play a role (Iskandrian et al. 1992). Figure 3.5 shows the variety of systolic blood pressure responses to aerobic exercise in patients with ischemic heart disease.

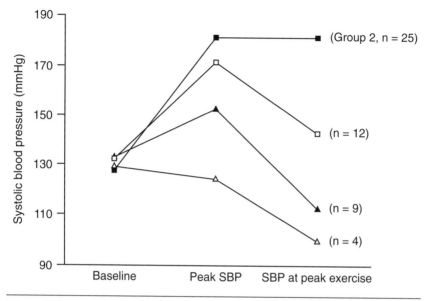

Figure 3.5   Various systolic blood pressure responses during graded exercise testing in patients with coronary artery disease.
Reprinted by permission of the publisher from Mechanism of exercise-induced hypotension in coronary artery disease by Iskandrian AS, Kegel JG, Lemlek J, Heo J, Cave V, Iskandrian B., *Am J Cardiol* 69, 1519. Copyright 1992 by Excerpta Medica Inc.

Diastolic hypertension (increase of 15 mmHg or greater during aerobic exercise) is associated with worsening left ventricular function during exercise (Paraskevaidis et al. 1993). Some patients exhibit an increase in systolic blood pressure during recovery from exercise rather than the normal decline in pressure (see figure 3.6). This paradoxical blood pressure response is associated with severe ischemia and an increase in postexercise stroke volume (Hashimoto et al. 1993).

Graded Exercise Testing in Myocardial Ischemia

Assessment of exercise capacity and the presence and extent of myocardial ischemia may be accomplished using several different techniques, including the following:

- Standard exercise electrocardiogram
- Nuclear imaging modalities
- Echocardiographic determination of ventricular systolic function and regional wall motion (stress echocardiography)

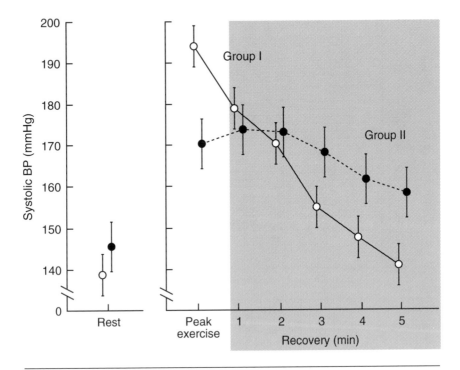

Figure 3.6   Recovery (post treadmill exercise testing) systolic blood pressure responses in patients with coronary artery disease. Group I patients exhibit the normal decline in systolic blood pressure while group II patients' blood pressures increased abnormally during recovery from exercise. Values are the mean ± SEM.

Reprinted from *The American Journal of Cardiology*, 76, Abe K, Tsuda M, Hayashi H, Hirai M, Sato A, Tsuzuki J, Saito H., Diagnostic usefulness of post-exercise systolic blood pressure response for detection of coronary artery disease in patients with electrocardiographic left ventricular hypertrophy, 893, Copyright 1995, with permission from Excerpta Medica Inc.

In any testing modality, the clinical interpretation of the test results requires integration of all of the available clinical data. These tests are not infallible in detecting the presence or absence of myocardial ischemia. An excellent discussion of test interpretation is provided by Ellestad (1996). A recent review from the Mayo Clinic provides a comparison of the various testing techniques (Mayo Clinic Cardiovascular Working Group on Stress Testing 1996).

Standard Exercise Electrocardiology

Standard exercise electrocardiography, with ST segment depression (or less commonly, ST segment elevation) of ≥ 1 mm at 0.08 seconds after the J point required for the diagnosis of ischemia, provides a sensitivity of approximately 65% to 70%. Other factors such as the time of onset of ST depression (early in exercise versus near-maximal exertion), the maximal amount of ST change, and the presence of typical angina increase the accuracy of the assessment of ischemia.

Limitations of the exercise ECG are its inability to diagnose ischemia in the setting of digoxin use or an abnormal rest ECG (particularly left bundle branch block), inability to localize the area of the myocardium that is ischemic by ST depression, lower sensitivity than with imaging techniques (sensitivities of 85%+), and the lack of information provided regarding the extent of ischemia. The exercise ECG does provide evidence of the ischemic threshold (the heart rate and systolic blood pressure that correspond to the first evidence of ischemia), which is valuable in prescribing physical activity for patients.

Nuclear Imaging Modalities

Myocardial perfusion imaging using radioisotopes (thallium and sestamibi) is based on the premise that myocardial uptake of these substances is proportional to myocardial blood flow. Images are obtained at rest and after exercise with a single photon emission computed tomography camera system. Reversible defects (better perfusion at rest than with exercise) represent ischemia. Fixed defects (present at rest and with exercise) represent infarct scar or, less commonly, stunned or hibernating myocardium. The images provide quantification of infarct size. Increased pulmonary uptake of thallium is a poor prognostic indicator.

Thallium-201 imaging is performed in two stages. First, exercise testing with immediate postexercise imaging is performed. Second, after a period of approximately three hours, redistribution imaging is performed, which allows differentiation of the presence of ischemia versus infarction. A second agent, $^{99\,m}$Tc sestamibi, experiences less soft tissue attenuation and results in higher resolution images, and is ideal for obese patients. The sestamibi technique also provides a resting first-pass measurement of left ventricular ejection fraction. The study is performed on two separate days. On the first day, rest images are obtained. Postmaximal exercise data is obtained on the second day and ischemia versus infarction may be delineated, as for thallium imaging. These perfusion imaging techniques do not provide evidence of the ischemic threshold.

Exercise radionuclide angiography (also termed radionuclide ventriculography, or multiple gated acquisition scanning [MUGA]) uses $^{99\,m}$Tc pertechnetate to form an intravascular blood pool image (an angiogram) and provides mechanical heart function information. Graded semisupine exercise is performed on a cycle ergometer with quantification of LVEF and ventricular volumes, and subjective assessment of regional wall motion at rest and for each exercise stage, thus providing evidence for the ischemic threshold. Myocardial ischemia is diagnosed if new regional wall-motion abnormalities occur, or if LVEF fails to increase or decreases during exercise. The heart rate and blood pressure responses to supine exercise are different than for upright exercise (Stenberg et al. 1967). Heart rates tend to be lower, and both systolic and diastolic blood pressures tend to be higher for supine than for upright exercise. Right ventricular size and function may also be evaluated with this technique. Exercise radionuclide angiography is inaccurate in diagnosing ischemia in the presence of an irregular rhythm (for example, atrial fibrillation) and resting regional wall-motion abnormalities.

Exercise Echocardiography

In exercise echocardiography, quantitative echo images of LVEF and end-systolic volume and subjective echo images of regional wall motion and thickening are obtained before and immediately after maximal exercise. Information regarding valvular function may also be obtained. As with radionuclide angiography, the diagnosis of ischemia is problematic in patients with resting regional wall-motion abnormalities. This technique does not provide serial information during graded exercise and does not provide information regarding the ischemic threshold.

Exercise for the various imaging techniques (with the exception of MUGA) is usually performed on a motorized treadmill, although cycle ergometry, or arm only, or combination arm and leg ergometry may be preferable in certain situations. Exercise testing protocols and procedures for patients with coronary artery disease are described in several excellent references (American College of Sports Medicine 1995; Ellestad 1996), and are not reviewed here.

Pharmacological Stress Testing

Pharmacological stress testing using intravenous administration of coronary vasodilators or positive chronotropic and inotropic agents may be used in conjunction with nuclear or echocardiographic imaging for patients who cannot exercise adequately. Dipyridamole and adenosine are coronary vasodilators that are commonly used with nuclear perfusion imaging techniques. An abnormal flow reserve (less flow in a particular region of the myocardium relative to other regions) in the territory supplied by a stenotic coronary artery represents an ischemic response. All of the exercise imaging techniques are inaccurate in the presence of left bundle branch block on the electrocardiogram. However, dipyridamole thallium perfusion imaging is useful in the presence of left bundle branch block. Dobutamine is a synthetic sympathomimetic that increases both myocardial contractility and heart rate, thus elevating myocardial oxygen requirement in a manner analogous to exercise. It is commonly used in conjunction with continuous echocardiographic assessment of ventricular function. At the maximum dose of dobutamine, if the heart rate is below 85% of age-predicted, atropine may be given to further increase the heart rate. With any of the techniques of assessing myocardial ischemia, the expertise and experience of the clinicians performing the tests are of paramount importance.

Acute Exercise Responses in Chronic Heart Failure

As discussed previously, exercise capacity for a given left ventricular ejection fraction is highly variable, although most patients with chronic heart failure have below normal aerobic capacities. It must be emphasized that resting LVEF does not predict exercise capacity.

$\dot{V}O_2$ peak and Ventilatory Anaerobic Threshold

Several investigators have demonstrated that $\dot{V}O_2$ peak is quite reproducible in heart failure patients (Janicki et al. 1990; Cohen-Solal et al. 1991; see figure 3.7). For patients with normal left ventricular ejection fractions and heart failure due to diastolic dysfunction, aerobic capacity is reduced to a degree similar to that of patients with systolic dysfunction (Kitzman et al. 1997; Kitzman et al. 1991).

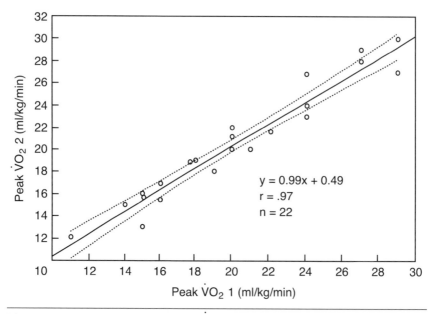

Figure 3.7   Reproducibility of peak $\dot{V}O_2$ for patients with chronic heart failure.
From *Eur Heart J*, 12, Cohen-Solal A, Zannad F, Kayanakis JG, Gueret P, Aupetit JF, Kolsky H., Multicentre study of the determination of peak oxygen uptake and ventilatory threshold during bicycle exercise in chronic heart failure: Comparison of graphical methods, interobserver variability and influence of the exercise protocol, 1055-1063, 1991, by permission of the publisher W B Saunders Company Limited London.

The ventilatory threshold, measured by a variety of techniques, is not as reproducible in heart failure patients as the $\dot{V}O_2$peak (Cohen-Solal et al. 1994; Cohen-Solal et al. 1991; see figure 3.8). In particular, the ventilatory threshold appears to be difficult to determine in patients with a $\dot{V}O_2$peak of 10 ml/kg/min or less (Katz et al. 1992). Therefore, $\dot{V}O_2$peak has become the accepted measure of exercise tolerance in patients with heart failure.

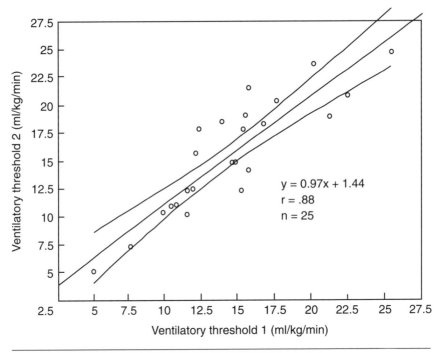

Figure 3.8 Reproducibility of the ventilatory threshold for patients with chronic heart failure.

Reprinted from *Eur Heart J*, 12, Cohen-Solal A, Zannad F, Kayanakis JG, Gueret P, Aupetit JF, Kolsky H., Multicentre study of the determination of peak oxygen uptake and ventilatory threshold during bicycle exercise in chronic heart failure: Comparison of graphical methods, interobserver variability and influence of the exercise protocol, 1055-1063, 1991, by permission of the publisher W B Saunders Company Limited London.

The symptomatic status of patients with heart failure is related to exercise capacity. Symptomatic patients, as a group, have lower aerobic capacities than asymptomatic individuals (Liang et al. 1992; see table 3.1). However, even patients with asymptomatic left ventricular dysfunction have below normal average $\dot{V}O_2$peaks. LeJemtel and colleagues (1994) reported a $\dot{V}O_2$peak of 22 ml/kg/min for patients with an average LVEF of 29% and no excessive dyspnea or fatigue, compared with 30 ml/kg/min for age-matched controls. Patients and controls achieved similar peak exercise

Table 3.1   Exercise Test Performance in Asymptomatic (n=164) and Symptomatic (n=20) Chronic Heart Failure Patients

	Asymptomatic	Symptomatic	p value
Exercise duration (sec)	842 ± 277	493 ± 160	< .001
$\dot{V}O_2$peak (ml/kg/min)	20 ± 6	13 ± 4	< .001
Anaerobic threshold (ml/kg/min)	16 ± 5	11 ± 4	< .001

Reprinted by permission of the publisher from Characteristics of peak aerobic capacity in symptomatic and asymptomatic subjects with left ventricular dysfunction by Liang C, Stewart DK, LeJemtel TH, Kirlin PC, McIntyre KM, Robertson T, Brown R, Moore AW, Wellington KL, Cahill L, Galvao M, Woods PA, Garces C, Held P., *Am J Cardiol* 69:1209. Copyright 1992 by Excerpta Medica Inc.

respiratory exchange ratios and ratings of perceived exertion consistent with near-maximal effort.

The New York Heart Association classification of symptomatic status does not predict exercise capacity accurately (Smith et al. 1993; see table 3.2). Weber and associates (1988) have proposed a classification system for the severity of heart failure based on $\dot{V}O_2$peak, as shown in table 3.3.

Weber et al. have shown that $\dot{V}O_2$peak is closely related to stroke volume index (see figure 3.9) and cardiac index (see figure 3.10) during maximal

Table 3.2   Relationship of New York Heart Association Class and $\dot{V}O_2$peak in 804 Patients With Left Ventricular Dysfunction

$\dot{V}O_2$peak (ml/kg/min)	NYHA Class I	II	III-IV	n
< 10	1 (1%)	29 (27%)	79 (72%)	109
≥ 10 to < 15	16 (4%)	223 (54%)	174 (42%)	413
≥ 15	29 (11%)	152 (56%)	92 (34%)	273

Reproduced, with permission, from Smith RF, Johnson G, Ziesche S, Bhat G, Blamkenship K, Cohn JN. Functional capacity in heart failure: Comparison of methods for assessment and their relation to other indexes of heart failure. *Circulation* 87:VI-18. Copyright 1993 American Heart Association.

Table 3.3   Weber Grading Scale of Chronic Heart Failure Severity by $\dot{V}O_2$peak

Class	Impairment	$\dot{V}O_2$peak (ml/kg/min)
A	Little or none	> 20
B	Mild to moderate	16-20
C	Moderate to severe	10-16
D	Severe	< 10

From Weber KT, et al.: Monitoring Physical Activity in Ambulatory Patients with Chronic Heart Failure in David, D et al (Eds), Ambulatory Monitoring of the Cardiac Patient (*Cardiovascular Clinics* 18/3), F.A. Davis Company, 1988.

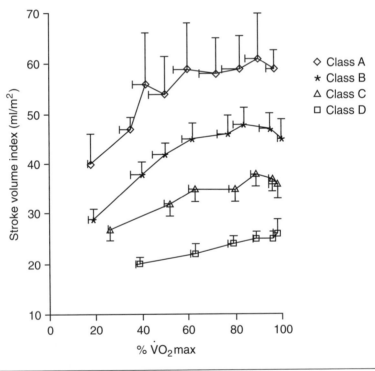

Figure 3.9   Stroke volume index response to incremental exercise in chronic heart failure patients with worsening $\dot{V}O_2$peak (A→D).

Reprinted, with permission, from Weber KT, Janicki JS, McElroy PA, Reddy HK. 1985. Monitoring physical activity in ambulatory patients with chronic heart failure. *Heart Failure 1:* 131. Copyright 1985 LeJacq Communications, Inc.

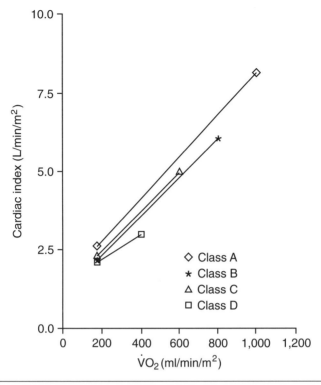

Figure 3.10   The relationship of cardiac index and oxygen uptake ($\dot{V}O_2$) for different functional classes of chronic heart failure.

Reprinted, with permission, from Weber KT, Janicki JS, McElroy PA, Reddy HK. 1985. Monitoring physical activity in ambulatory patients with chronic heart failure. *Heart Failure 1:* 131. Copyright 1985 LeJacq Communications, Inc.

tolerated exercise. Figure 3.11 gives the relationships among Weber functional class, cardiac index, and pulmonary capillary wedge pressure. With worsening heart failure class based upon $\dot{V}O_2$peak, cardiac index is lower and wedge pressure is higher. Thus, the Weber classification system appears to be a valid marker for heart failure severity and is well accepted.

$\dot{V}O_2$ Kinetics

Many patients with left ventricular dysfunction demonstrate abnormally long $\dot{V}O_2$ kinetics at both the onset (Sietsema et al. 1994; Koike et al. 1995; Riley et al. 1994; Zhang et al. 1993) and offset (Hayashida et al. 1993; Cohen-Solal et al. 1995) of exercise. This explains the inaccuracy (overestimation) of indirect estimates of oxygen uptake based on treadmill or cycle external workload. Some patients with more severe heart failure may demonstrate

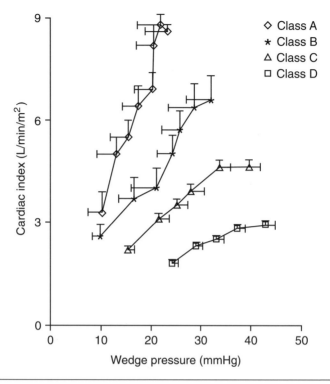

Figure 3.11   The response of the cardiac index and pulmonary capillary wedge pressure to incremental exercise for each Weber functional class.

Reprinted, with permission, from Weber KT, Janicki JS, McElroy PA, Reddy HK. 1985. Monitoring physical activity in ambulatory patients with chronic heart failure. *Heart Failure 1:* 131. Copyright 1985 LeJacq Communications, Inc.

a characteristic plateau or further increase in $\dot{V}O_2$ during the early recovery phase of a maximal graded exercise test (Daida et al. 1996). Figure 3.12 provides an example of this phenomenon compared with the usual rapid decline in $\dot{V}O_2$ during the early recovery phase. For a given absolute submaximal exercise intensity, the time for development of a steady state $\dot{V}O_2$ is delayed for heart failure patients, resulting in a larger oxygen deficit and increased reliance on anaerobic energy production at the onset of exercise (Cross and Higginbotham 1995; see figure 3.13). For example, Sietsema et al. (1994) reported that for a cycle exercise intensity of 25 watts, normal control subjects exhibited a mean $\dot{V}O_2$ response time of approximately 37 seconds for the achievement of a steady state. Patients with heart failure required 67 seconds for mean response time. With worsening of heart failure, $\dot{V}O_2$ kinetics progressively lengthen. Koike and colleagues (1994) have demonstrated more prolonged $\dot{V}O_2$ kinetics for patients with heart failure who have lower left ventricular ejection fractions (30%) than

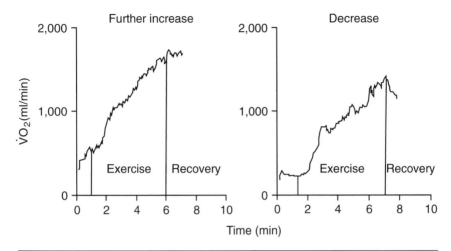

Figure 3.12 Example of $\dot{V}O_2$ kinetics with (left) or without (right) a further increase in $\dot{V}O_2$ during recovery in patients with chronic heart failure. The normal response is shown on the right. On the left, $\dot{V}O_2$ was $\geq \dot{V}O_2$peak during the first 30 seconds of active recovery.

Reprinted, with permission, from Daida H, Allison TG, Johnson BD, Squires RW, Gau GT. 1996. Further increase in oxygen uptake during early active recovery following maximal exercise in chronic heart failure. *Chest* 109:47-51.

for patients with the same $\dot{V}O_2$peak with higher ejection fractions (39%), as seen in figure 3.14.

In addition, Cohen-Solal and colleagues (1990) have demonstrated a lower change in $\dot{V}O_2$ per increase in cycle ergometer exercise intensity with worsening Weber class (see table 3.4). Figure 3.15 provides a graphic display of the progressively lower $\dot{V}O_2$ during incremental cycle exercise for normal controls and Weber classes A-D. A substantially lower submaximal $\dot{V}O_2$ is seen for classes B-D compared to normal controls and class A heart failure patients.

As mentioned above, at the completion of exercise the offset $\dot{V}O_2$ kinetics are also prolonged for many heart failure patients compared to controls. Figure 3.16 shows the difference between the half-time of recovery of $\dot{V}O_2$ for a normal control individual and a CHF patient. Hayashida et al. (1993) have reported time constants for recovery $\dot{V}O_2$ kinetics after peak exercise of 118 seconds and 169 seconds for a normal person and an age-matched patient with dilated cardiomyopathy, respectively.

Hemodynamic Responses

Sullivan and associates (1989), in an elegant investigation, studied the central hemodynamic responses to upright graded cycle exercise to exhaustion in 30 patients with chronic heart failure (22 with coronary artery

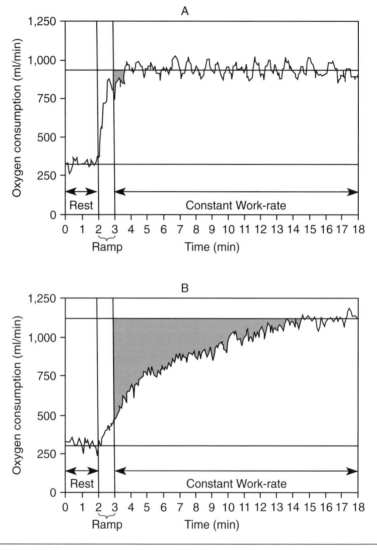

Figure 3.13 Oxygen consumption during 15 minutes of cycle exercise at 25 watts. The shaded area represents the oxygen deficit. A = control subject, B = chronic heart failure patient.

Reprinted, with permission, from Cross AM, Higginbotham MB. 1995. Oxygen deficit during exercise testing in heart failure: Relation to submaximal exercise tolerance. *Chest* 107:904-908.

disease, eight with dilated cardiomyopathy (mean left ventricular ejection fraction 24%, range 8% to 36%) and 12 healthy control subjects. Oxygen uptake was measured directly and the subjects were instrumented as follows: Swan-Ganz catheter in the right pulmonary artery, catheters in the

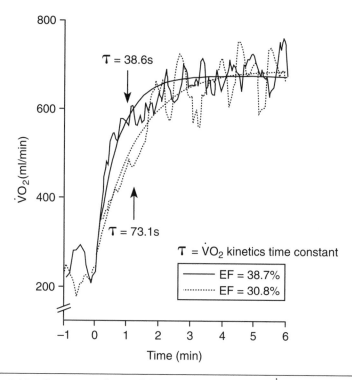

Figure 3.14   Computer-derived line of best fit of the $\dot{V}O_2$ response in two patients with chronic heart failure. The $\dot{V}O_2$ kinetics time constant was longer (slower kinetics) for the patient with the lower left ventricular ejection fraction (EF).

Reproduced, with permission, from Koike A, Hiroe M, Adachi H, Yajima T, Yamauchi Y, Nogami A, Ito H, Miyahara Y, Korenaga M, Marumo F. Oxygen uptake kinetics are determined by cardiac function at onset of exercise rather than peak exercise in patients with prior myocardial infarction. *Circulation* 90:2329. Copyright 1994 American Heart Association.

femoral vein and brachial artery, and a femoral vein thermodilution catheter for leg blood flow measurements. As expected, $\dot{V}O_2$peak was lower for patients than controls (15.1 ± 4.8 versus 32.1 ± 9.9 ml/kg/min, p < .001). Serial measurements of heart rate, stroke volume, cardiac output, and arterial-mixed venous oxygen difference are given in figure 3.17.

Submaximal exercise heart rates were consistently higher for patients, although peak exercise heart rate was substantially lower than controls. Stroke volume and cardiac output were also lower for patients during submaximal and maximal exercise. An interesting compensatory elevation in arterial-mixed venous oxygen difference during submaximal exercise intensities was seen in the chronic heart failure patients. Figure 3.18 shows that the larger arterial-mixed venous oxygen difference in the patients

Table 3.4   Change in $\dot{V}O_2$ per Change in Cycle Exercise Intensity in Watts ($\Delta\dot{V}O_2/\Delta W$) for Normal Controls (n=27) and Chronic Heart Failure Patients, Weber Class A to D (n=77)

	$\Delta\dot{V}O_2/\Delta W$ (ml/min/watt)
Controls	11.05 ± 0.38
Class A	11.44 ± 1.48
Class B	10.05 ± 1.61
Class C-D	8.75 ± 2.14*
All classes	10.22 ± 2.04

Reprinted from *Journal of the American College of Cardiology*, 16, Cohen-Solal A, Chabernaud JM, Gourgon R., Comparison of oxygen uptake during bicycle exercise in patients with chronic heart failure and in normal subjects, 82, Copyright 1990, with permission from the American College of Cardiology.

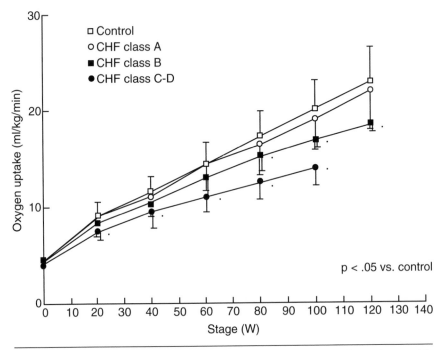

Figure 3.15   Oxygen uptake during graded cycle ergometry in patients with worsening degrees of heart failure (Weber class A-D) and control subjects. $\dot{V}O_2$ becomes lower as the severity of heart failure worsens.

Reprinted from *The American Journal of Cardiology*, 67, Cohen-Solal A, Gourgon R., Assessment of exercise tolerance in chronic congestive heart failure, 38C, Copyright 1991, with permission from Excerpta Medica Inc.

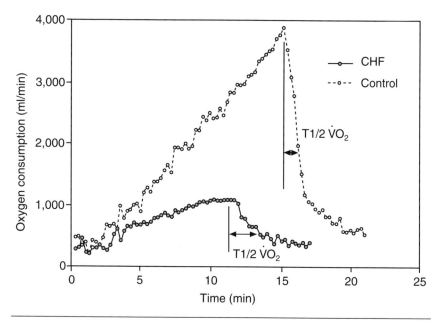

Figure 3.16 Example of recovery of oxygen consumption after exercise in a control subject and a patient with chronic heart failure (CHF). The half-time of recovery of oxygen consumption ($_{t1/2}\dot{V}O_2$) is the time between $\dot{V}O_2$peak and 50% of $\dot{V}O_2$peak at recovery.

Reproduced, with permission, from Cohen-Solal A, Laperche T, Morvan D, Geneves M, Caviezel B, Gourgon R. Prolonged kinetics of recovery of oxygen consumption after maximal graded exercise in patients with chronic heart failure: Analysis with gas exchange measurements and NMR spectroscopy. *Circulation* 91:2926. Copyright 1995 American Heart Association.

resulted in a normal increase in $\dot{V}O_2$ during the early stages of graded exercise. Mean arterial pressure was well maintained in patients throughout exercise by an elevated systemic vascular resistance (see figure 3.19), in spite of the subnormal cardiac output response. This is consistent with a reflex-mediated relative peripheral vasoconstriction to maintain blood pressure during exercise. Pulmonary vascular resistance and pulmonary capillary wedge pressure were also higher throughout all stages of exercise in patients compared with controls.

Notwithstanding the normal mean exercise systemic blood pressure, exercise leg blood flow is reduced in the patients, due, in part, to an elevated leg vascular resistance (see figure 3.20). Leg arterial-mixed venous oxygen difference is somewhat elevated in the patients, but this provides only a partial compensation as leg $\dot{V}O_2$ lags behind that of the controls after only the second exercise stage (see figure 3.21). Figure 3.22 shows the strong, positive relationship between $\dot{V}O_2$peak and peak exercise cardiac output

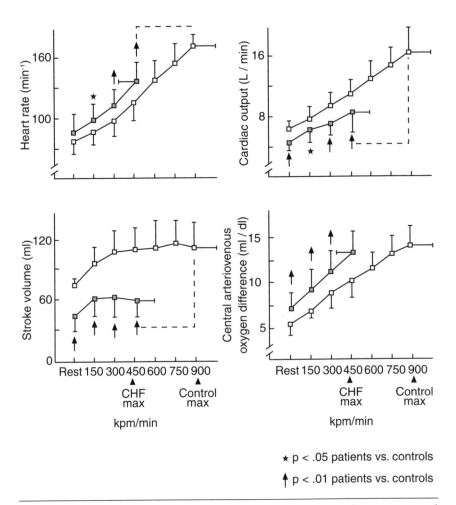

Figure 3.17   Rest and exercise heart rate, stroke volume, cardiac output, and central arteriovenous oxygen difference in patients with chronic heart failure (■) and control subjects (□).

Reproduced, with permission, from Sullivan MJ, Knight JD, Higginbotham MB, Cobb FR. Relation between central and peripheral hemodynamics during exercise in patients with chronic heart failure: Muscle blood flow is reduced with maintenance of arterial perfusion pressure. *Circulation* 80:773. Copyright 1989 American Heart Association.

and leg blood flow. This relationship has been reported by other investigators. For example, Metra and colleagues (1990) reported a correlation of .89 between cardiac index and $\dot{V}O_2$peak in a group of 34 chronic heart failure patients.

Roubin and coworkers (1990) replicated the study of Sullivan with nearly identical results in a group of 23 patients (10 with coronary artery disease,

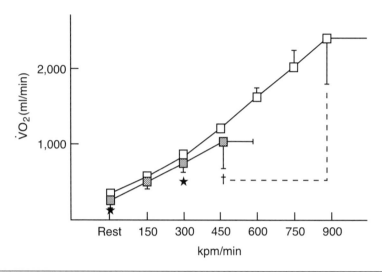

Figure 3.18   Rest and exercise (cycle ergometry in kpm/min) $\dot{V}O_2$ in patients with chronic heart failure (▨) and control subjects (□). ★ p < .05, † p < .01.

Reproduced, with permission, from Sullivan MJ, Knight JD, Higginbotham MB, Cobb FR. Relation between central and peripheral hemodynamics during exercise in patients with chronic heart failure: Muscle blood flow is reduced with maintenance of arterial perfusion pressure. *Circulation* 80:772. Copyright 1989 American Heart Association.

13 with dilated cardiomyopathy) with mean left ventricular ejection fractions of 24% and $\dot{V}O_2$ peaks of approximately 15 ml/kg/min. Subjects in this investigation were also studied with gated radionuclide angiography and demonstrated a flat left ventricular ejection response to graded exercise (see figure 3.23).

During upright exercise, however, end-diastolic volume does increase in some patients with chronic heart failure. This allows the Frank-Starling mechanism to operate resulting in an increase in stroke volume with a flat left ventricular ejection fraction response (Tomai et al. 1993; see figure 3.24). Dahan et al. (1995) have reported the importance of preload reserve, or the ability of the heart with systolic dysfunction to dilate, in determining the stroke volume response to exercise. Figure 3.25 shows the relationship of a global index of left ventricular distensibility to exercise capacity. Abnormal left ventricular distensibility is common in patients with ischemic left ventricular systolic dysfunction (Pouleur et al. 1990).

It should be pointed out that some investigators have found variable central hemodynamic responses to graded exercise in some chronic heart failure patients. Hecht et al. (1982) reported that, in a group of 13 patients with similar exercise capacities, some patients increased cardiac index and stroke volume index while other patients demonstrated a markedly blunted hemodynamic response (see figure 3.26). Similarly, Wilson and colleagues

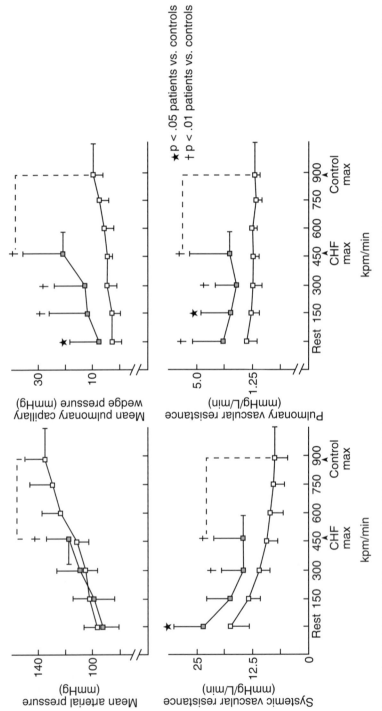

Figure 3.19 Rest and exercise mean arterial pressure and systemic vascular resistance in patients with chronic heart failure (■) and control subjects (□).

Reproduced, with permission, from Sullivan MJ, Knight JD, Higginbotham MB, Cobb FR. Relation between central and peripheral hemodynamics during exercise in patients with chronic heart failure: Muscle blood flow is reduced with maintenance of arterial perfusion pressure. *Circulation* 80:774. Copyright 1989 American Heart Association.

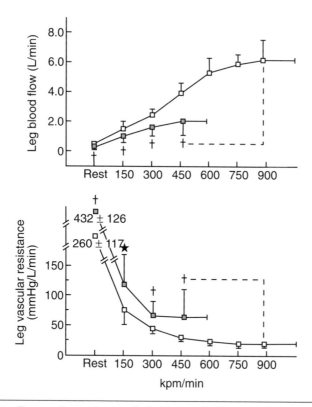

Figure 3.20   Rest and exercise single leg blood flow and vascular resistance in patients with chronic heart failure (■) and control subjects (□). ★ p < .05, † p < .01.

Reproduced, with permission, from Sullivan MJ, Knight JD, Higginbotham MB, Cobb FR. Relation between central and peripheral hemodynamics during exercise in patients with chronic heart failure: Muscle blood flow is reduced with maintenance of arterial perfusion pressure. *Circulation* 80:774. Copyright 1989 American Heart Association.

(1995) reported a poor relationship between cardiac index and $\dot{V}O_2$peak (see figure 3.27) in a population of patients with severe exercise impairment (mean $\dot{V}O_2$peak of 13 ml/kg/min). However, Cohen-Solal and associates (1996) demonstrated that during graded exercise in heart failure patients, an abrupt decrease in cardiac output due, for example, to the onset of rapid atrial fibrillation or third degree heart block results in an immediate decrease in $\dot{V}O_2$.

Responses to Arm Exercise

Keteyian and colleagues (1996) compared the responses to graded arm crank and leg cycle exercise of 20 heart failure patients (mean LVEF 23 ± 8%) and 10 age-matched healthy control subjects. The $\dot{V}O_2$ peak for arm exercise

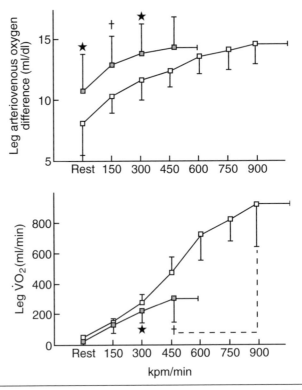

Figure 3.21 Rest and exercise single leg arteriovenous oxygen difference and $\dot{V}O_2$ in patients with chronic heart failure (■) and control subjects (□). ★ p < .05, † p < .01.

Reproduced, with permission, from Sullivan MJ, Knight JD, Higginbotham MB, Cobb FR. Relation between central and peripheral hemodynamics during exercise in patients with chronic heart failure: Muscle blood flow is reduced with maintenance of arterial perfusion pressure. *Circulation* 80:774. Copyright 1989 American Heart Association.

in heart failure patients averaged 12 ml/kg/min versus 16 ml/kg/min for controls (63% of controls). For leg cycling, $\dot{V}O_2$peak was 19 ml/kg/min and 29 ml/kg/min for heart failure and control subjects, respectively (55% of controls). For a given power output, $\dot{V}O_2$ was higher for arm exercise than leg exercise, as expected, for both patients and controls. Peak arm exercise responses were similar for both groups when expressed as a percentage of peak leg exercise responses (see table 3.5).

Heart Rate

The heart rate response to graded exercise is variable in patients with left ventricular dysfunction. Figure 3.28 shows the progressive chronotropic incompetence in patients with worsening Weber class (Colucci et al. 1989). Heart rate and blood pressure at peak exercise are lower, on average, for

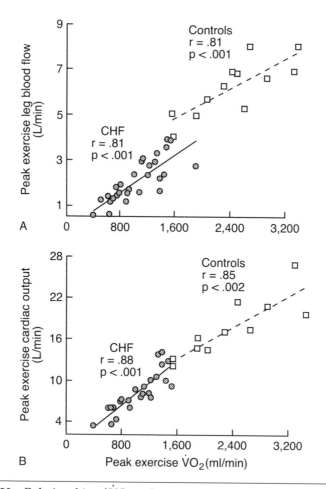

Figure 3.22   Relationship of $\dot{V}O_2$peak to single leg blood flow (A) and cardiac output (B) in patients with chronic heart failure (◉) and control subjects (□).

Reproduced, with permission, from Sullivan MJ, Knight JD, Higginbotham MB, Cobb FR. Relation between central and peripheral hemodynamics during exercise in patients with chronic heart failure: Muscle blood flow is reduced with maintenance of arterial perfusion pressure. *Circulation* 80:778. Copyright 1989 American Heart Association.

patients with more compromised exercise capacities (see table 3.6). Heart failure may result in decreased cardiac responsiveness to sympathetic nervous system stimulation during exercise (Rundquist et al. 1997).

Skeletal Muscle Blood Flow

With worsening heart failure, as determined by $\dot{V}O_2$peak, nutritive blood flow to the leg skeletal muscle becomes progressively impaired (Wilson et al. 1984b). This is graphically illustrated in figure 3.29. Reduced leg blood

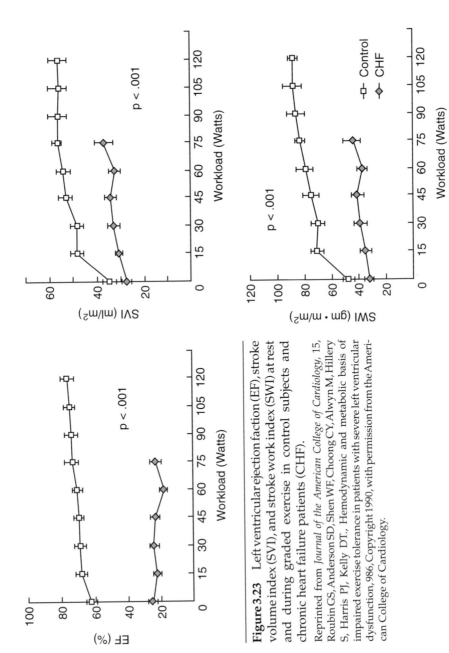

Figure 3.23 Left ventricular ejection faction (EF), stroke volume index (SVI), and stroke work index (SWI) at rest and during graded exercise in control subjects and chronic heart failure patients (CHF).

Reprinted from *Journal of the American College of Cardiology*, 15, Roubin GS, Anderson SD, Shen WF, Choong CY, Alwyn M, Hillery S, Harris PJ, Kelly DT., Hemodynamic and metabolic basis of impaired exercise tolerance in patients with severe left ventricular dysfunction, 986, Copyright 1990, with permission from the American College of Cardiology.

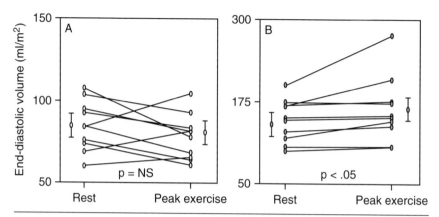

Figure 3.24 Changes in left ventricular end-diastolic volume from rest to peak exercise in control subjects (A) and in patients with dilated cardiomyopathy (B).

Reprinted from *The American Journal of Cardiology*, 72, Tomai F, Ciavolella M, Cren F, Gaspardone A, Versaci F, Giannitti C, Scali D, Chiariello L, Gioffre PA., Left ventricular volumes during exercise in normal subjects and patients with dilated cardiomyopathy assessed by first-pass radionuclide angiography, 1169, Copyright 1993, with permission from Excerpta Medica Inc.

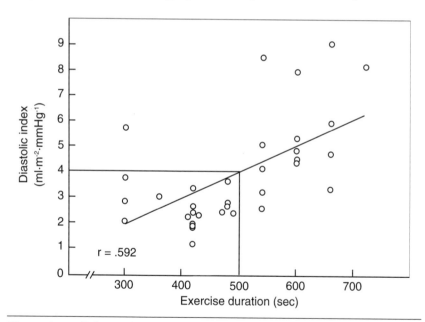

Figure 3.25 Relationship of exercise duration (graded exercise test) and a global measure of left ventricular diastolic distensibility (diastolic filling volume/mean left ventricular pressure during filling) in patients with left ventricular dysfunction.

Reproduced, with permission, from Pouleur H, Hanet C, Rousseau MF, VanEyll C. Relation of diastolic function and exercise capacity in ischemic left ventricular dysfunction: Role of β-agonists and β-antiagonists. *Circulation* 82:I-92. Copyright 1990 American Heart Association.

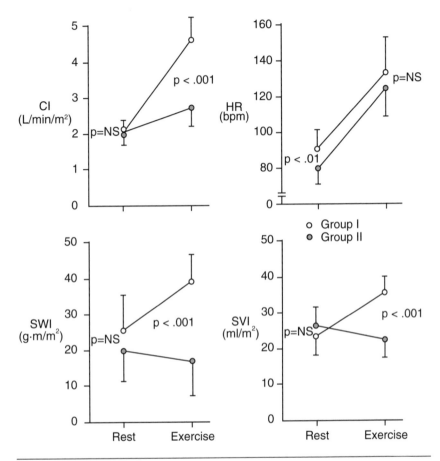

Figure 3.26 Comparison of patients with chronic heart failure with a normal (Group I) or abnormal (Group II) cardiac index (CI), stroke work index (SWI), and stroke volume index (SVI) response to exercise. Heart rate (HR) responses were similar for the two groups.

Reprinted, with permission, from Hecht HS, Karahalios SE, Ormiston JA, Schnugg SJ, Hopkins JM, Singh BN. 1982. Patterns of exercise response in patients with severe left ventricular dysfunction: Radionuclide ejection fraction and hemodynamic cardiac performance evaluations. *Am Heart J* 104:718-724.

flows are associated with lower aerobic capacities, implying a progressive impairment of skeletal muscle vasodilation during exercise.

Reading and associates (1993) demonstrated a reduction in calf blood flow during rhythmic plantar and dorsiflexion in patients with chronic heart failure. Calf vascular conductance (ml/min local flow per 10 L of tissue per mmHg), in their experiment, was 40.7 ± 4.3 versus 30.7 ± 6.1 for normal controls and CHF patients, respectively (p < .01). It appears that

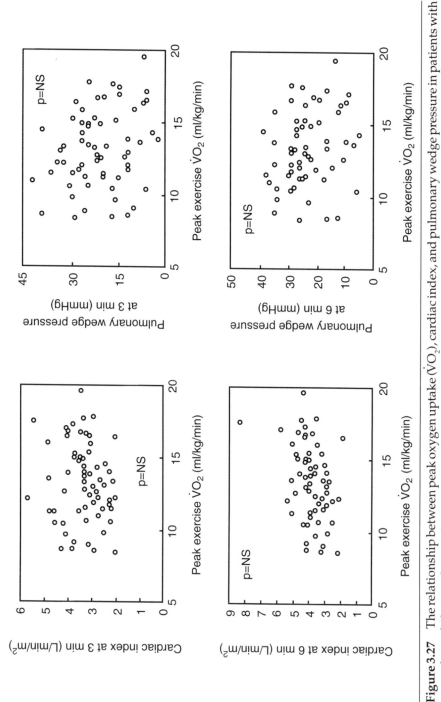

Figure 3.27 The relationship between peak oxygen uptake ($\dot{V}O_2$), cardiac index, and pulmonary wedge pressure in patients with severe heart failure at three and six minutes of exercise.

Reprinted from *Journal of the American College of Cardiology, 26*, Wilson JR, Rayos G, Yeoh TK, Gothard P., Dissociation between peak exercise oxygen consumption and hemodynamic dysfunction in potential heart transplant candidates, 432, Copyright 1995, with permission from the American College of Cardiology.

Table 3.5 Peak Arm Cranking Exercise Responses for Heart Failure Patients and Healthy Controls Expressed as the Percentage of Peak Leg Cycling Responses

	Heart failure patients	Healthy controls
Power	43 ± 10	32 ± 9
Heart rate	89 ± 7	92 ± 9
$\dot{V}O_2$	74 ± 9	67 ± 12
Rate-pressure product	85 ± 14	89 ± 13

Reprinted, by permission, from Keteyian SJ, Marks CRC, Brawner CA, Levine AB, Kataoka T, Levine TB. 1996. Responses to arm exercise in patients with compensated heart failure. *J. Cardiopulmonary Rehabil* 16:366-371. Copyright 1996 Lippincott-Raven.

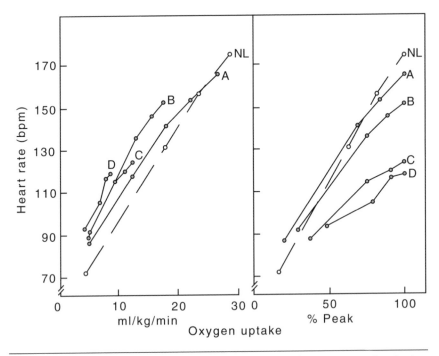

Figure 3.28 The relationship between heart rate and oxygen uptake during exercise in normal control subjects (NL) and patients with progressively more severe chronic heart failure classified by Weber criteria A, B, C, D.

Reproduced, with permission, from Colucci WS, Riberio JP, Rocco MB, Quigg RJ, Creager MA, Marsh JD, Gauthier DF, Hartley LF. Impaired chronotropic response to exercise in patients with congestive heart failure: Role of postsynaptic β-adrenergic desensitization. *Circulation* 80:317. Copyright 1989 American Heart Association.

Table 3.6   Relationship of Mean Peak Exercise Heart Rate (beats/ min ± SD) and Peak Oxygen Uptake in 804 Chronic Heart Failure Patients With Various Left Ventricular Ejection Fractions

| | $\dot{V}O_2$peak (ml/kg/min) | | | |
	≤ 10	> 10 to ≤ 15	> 15	p value
LVEF ≤ 25%	113.6 ± 16.6	128.9 ± 18.4	141.7 ± 21.4	< .001
LVEF > 25 to ≤ 35%	111.5 ± 14.2	126.3 ± 21.4	137.8 ± 22.4	< .001
LVEF > 35%	117.1 ± 29.9	119.9 ± 20.1	135.4 ± 21.4	< .001

Reproduced, with permission, from Smith RF, Johnson G, Ziesche S, Bhat G, Blamkenship K, Cohn JN. Functional capacity in heart failure: Comparison of methods for assessment and their relation to other indexes of heart failure. *Circulation* 87:VI-92. Copyright 1993 American Heart Association.

smaller muscle groups may be less affected by the reduction in blood flow during exercise than larger muscle groups. For example, peak hyperemic blood flow in the calf muscle has been shown to be reduced in CHF patients, although forearm flow after temporary arterial occlusion or submaximal isometric exercise is normal (Arnold et al. 1990; Jondeau et al. 1993). Figure 3.30 illustrates the finding of reduced hyperemic flow in calf muscle. It appears that the observed lower skeletal muscle blood flow is not simply due to a subnormal cardiac output because treatment with drugs such as dobutamine or cardiac transplantation, which immediately increase cardiac output, do not necessarily improve exercise capacity immediately (Wilson et al. 1984a; Muller et al. 1992). Some data suggest that nitric oxide-mediated exercise vasodilation is impaired in CHF patients (Katz et al. 1996).

Blood Lactate Concentration

At peak exercise, venous blood concentrations of lactate, glucose, and free fatty acids are similar in chronic heart failure patients and controls (Riley et al. 1993). However, as figure 3.31 shows, lactate accumulation in arterial blood, skeletal muscle, femoral venous blood, and the muscle-to-arterial blood lactate gradient occur earlier during graded exercise testing in heart failure patients than in healthy persons (Sullivan et al. 1991).

Riley and coworkers (1990) studied substrate utilization during 20 minutes of treadmill walking at an intensity of approximately 55% of $\dot{V}O_2$peak (below the ventilatory threshold) in a group of heart failure patients and controls. Figure 3.32 shows a higher venous blood lactate concentration during the entire exercise bout for heart failure patients; figure 3.33 illustrates the patients' propensity for heightened fat metabolism during exercise with elevated levels of plasma norepinephrine, serum

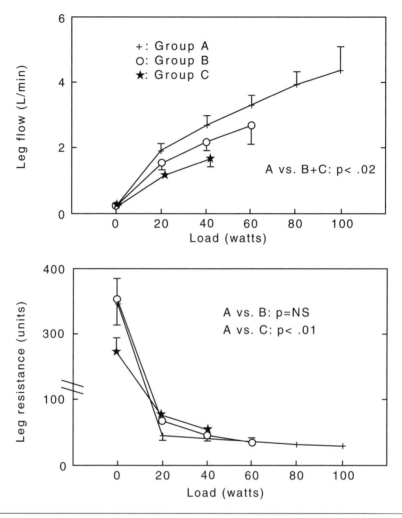

Figure 3.29 Leg blood flow and leg vascular resistance versus cycle exercise intensity for three groups of patients with chronic heart failure stratified by $\dot{V}O_2$peak (A: > 20 ml/kg/min, B: 15-18 ml/kg/min, C: < 14 ml/kg/min). Values are means ± SEM.

glycerol, serum hydroxybutyrate, and serum free fatty acids. The heavy reliance on fat as an energy source during moderate intensity exercise in chronic heart failure may represent a compensatory mechanism to conserve carbohydrate, but because fat is less efficient in the production of ATP

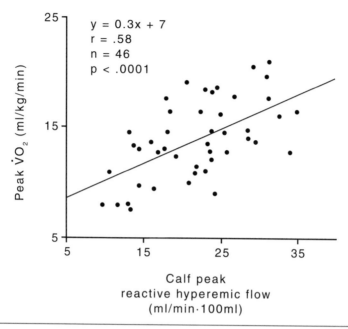

Figure 3.30   Calf peak reactive hyperemic blood flow induced by five minutes of arterial occlusion is linearly related to peak oxygen uptake ($\dot{V}O_2$) in 46 patients with chronic heart failure.

Reprinted from *Journal of the American College of Cardiology*, 22, Jondeau G, Katz SD, Toussaint JF, Dubourg O, Monrad ES, Bourdarias JP. LeJemtel TH., Regional specificity of peak hyperemic response in patients with congestive heart failure: Correlation with peak aerobic capacity, 1401, Copyright 1993, with permission from the American College of Cardiology.

(fewer ATP produced per L of O_2 consumed than with carbohydrate), this phenomenon may further impair exercise capacity.

High-Energy Phosphate Energetics

During exercise in heart failure, muscle high-energy phosphate energetics are also deranged. Studies using ^{31}P nuclear magnetic resonance during repetitive contraction of either the calf or finger flexors have demonstrated an earlier depletion of creatine phosphate in CHF patients than in control subjects (Massie et al. 1987; Massie et al. 1988; Marie et al. 1990; see figure 3.34) during both aerobic and ischemic (cuff arterial occlusion) exercise. This finding is consistent with a muscle metabolic abnormality that is independent of the reduced skeletal muscle blood flow during exercise discussed previously. The rate of mitochondrial ATP synthesis is decreased in CHF patients (Kemp et al. 1996). These data, in summary, demonstrate the above normal reliance on anaerobic energy production during even moderate intensity exercise in chronic heart failure.

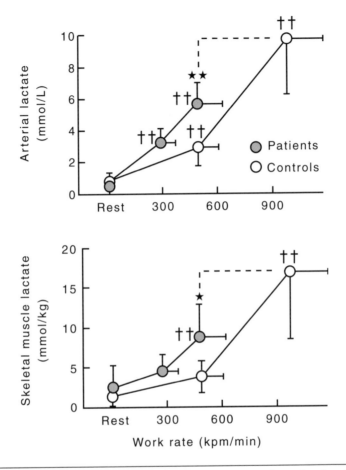

Figure 3.31   Arterial lactate content at rest and during submaximal and maximal exercise in chronic heart failure and control subjects (★★ p < .01 heart failure vs. control subjects; †† p < .01 vs. rest; ★ p < .05 patients vs. controls; † p < .05 vs. rest.)

Reproduced, with permission, from Sullivan MJ, Green HJ, Cobb FR. Altered skeletal muscle metabolic response to exercise in chronic heart failure: Relation to skeletal muscle aerobic enzyme activity. *Circulation* 84:1602. Copyright 1991 American Heart Association.

Skeletal Muscle Strength and Endurance

Several investigators, using either nuclear magnetic resonance imaging or electron beam computed tomography, have demonstrated a reduction in skeletal muscle mass of the quadriceps in patients with chronic heart failure, compared with size-matched controls (Minotti et al. 1993; Magnusson et al. 1994; Volterrani et al. 1994). Studies have reported either normal or impaired isokinetic strength in heart failure patients relative to healthy subjects. However, a substantial reduction in muscle endurance has been a consistent

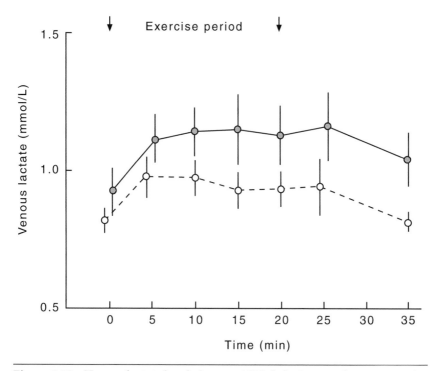

Figure 3.32 Venous lactate levels (means ± SEM) during steady state exercise in chronic heart failure patients (⦿-⦿) and normal controls (○-○). Lactate was significantly greater (p < .05) in patients.

Reprinted, with permission, from Riley M, Elborn JS, Bell N, Stanford CF, Nicholls DP. 1990. Substrate utilization during exercise in chronic cardiac failure. *Clin Sci* 79:89-95. Copyright 1990 The Biochemical Society and Medical Research Society.

finding (Minotti et al. 1991; Buller et al. 1991). Magnusson and coworkers (1994) reported that the remaining capacity to develop force after 50 maximal knee extensions was markedly impaired in heart failure patients (42% of 94±24 Nm) compared to controls (60% of 116±10 Nm). Heart failure patients also have a slower recovery of endurance after repetitive exercise (62 ± 4% for CHF patients versus 87 ± 7% for controls at five minutes) (Yamani et al. 1995). However, muscular endurance was fully restored in chronic heart failure patients after ten minutes of rest.

Breathing Responses

Breathing responses to exercise may be abnormal and unusual in patients with chronic heart failure. Standard measures of pulmonary function (forced expiratory volume in one second [FEV_1], forced vital capacity, diffusing capacity for carbon monoxide) are mildly depressed, as shown in table 3.7 (Kraemer et al. 1993). Mild bronchoconstriction may be present at

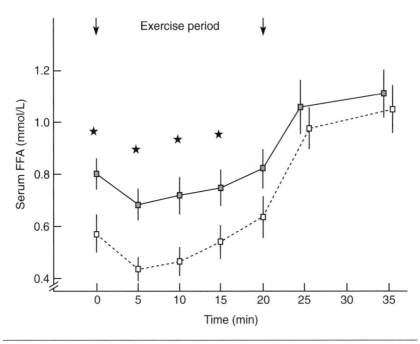

Figure 3.33   Serum free fatty acid (FFA) concentrations during steady state exercise (mean ± SEM) in chronic heart failure (■-■) and control subjects (□-□) (★ p < .05).

Reprinted, with permission, from Riley M, Elborn JS, Bell N, Stanford CF, Nicholls DP. 1990. Substrate utilization during exercise in chronic cardiac failure. *Clin Sci* 79:89-95. Copyright 1990 The Biochemical Society and Medical Research Society.

rest with improvement in FEV_1 (2.28-2.38 L) and $\dot{V}O_2$peak (16.3-17.9 ml/kg/min) with an inhaled bronchodilator (Uren et al. 1993b).

In spite of the mild reduction in diffusing capacity in heart failure, arterial blood gases and arterial oxygen saturation are normal during maximal exercise in most patients with compensated heart failure (Clark and Coats 1994; Messner-Pellenc et al. 1995). Clark and Coats (1994) studied 37 chronic heart failure patients during graded exercise with arterial blood gas sampling. Thirty-four patients had normal blood gas findings. The three patients with a decreased PO_2 during exercise all had alternative diagnoses for their desaturations (patent foramen ovale with a right to left shunt, pulmonary embolus, chronic obstructive lung disease). Arterial desaturation during exercise in patients with left ventricular dysfunction suggests a mechanism other than heart failure for the abnormality in blood gases.

McParland et al. (1992) measured maximal inspiratory and expiratory mouth pressures as indices of respiratory muscle strength in patients with left ventricular dysfunction. Some patients with chronic heart failure exhibited below normal respiratory muscle strength with a strong correlation

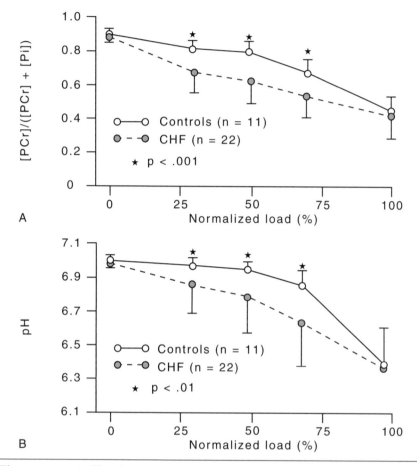

Figure 3.34   A. The change in the normalized phosphocreatine ratio during exercise relative to normalized exercise load in chronic heart failure (CHF) and control subjects. B. The change in pH relative to the normalized exercise load. PCr = phosphocreatine. Pi = inorganic phosphate.

Reproduced, with permission, from Massie B, Conway M, Yonge R, Frostick S, Ledingham J, Sleight P, Radda G, Rajagopalan B. Skeletal muscle metabolism in patients with congestive heart failure: Relation to clinical severity and blood flow. *Circulation* 76:1013. Copyright 1987 American Heart Association.

between dyspnea experienced during daily activities and respiratory muscle weakness. Acute unloading of the work of breathing during exercise by breathing a 79% helium/21% oxygen mixture improves exercise tolerance and makes breathing subjectively easier in heart failure patients but not in healthy control subjects (Mancini et al. 1997).

Uren and colleagues (1993a) presented evidence of a ventilation-perfusion mismatch in heart failure, with a slight improvement during exercise

Table 3.7   Pulmonary Function Variables for 50 Patients With Stable Chronic Heart Failure Compared to Predicted Values

		p value
FEV$_1$ (% predicted)	85 ± 16	< .01
FVC (% predicted)	89 ± 18	< .01
DLCO (% predicted)	81 ± 22	< .01

FEV$_1$ = forced expiratory volume in 1 second; FVC = forced vital capacity; DLCO = diffusing capacity for carbon monoxide.

Reprinted from *Journal of the American College of Cardiology*, 21, Kraemer MD, Kubo SH, Rector TS, Brunsvold N, Bank AJ., Pulmonary and peripheral vascular factors are important determinants of peak oxygen uptake in patients with heart failure, 644, Copyright 1993, with permission from the American College of Cardiology.

(see figure 3.35). As a result of this mismatch, a common finding in patients with left ventricular dysfunction during exercise is an excess ventilation, indicated by elevated ventilatory equivalents for O_2 (Myers et al. 1992; see figure 3.36) and CO_2 (see figure 3.37; Sovijarvi et al. 1992). During graded exercise, the ventilatory equivalent for CO_2 ($\dot{V}_E/\dot{V}CO_2$) decreases early in exercise and rises slightly at intensities above the ventilatory threshold. Failure of $\dot{V}_E/\dot{V}CO_2$ to decrease < 10% during early exercise is associated with more severe heart failure with an average $\dot{V}O_2$ peak of < 14 ml/kg/min (Milani et al. 1996).

The excess ventilation during exercise increases with severity of failure (Buller and Poole-Wilson 1990), and is not related to pulmonary hypertension in compensated heart failure (Davies et al. 1991). Figure 3.38 shows that the peak exercise pulmonary capillary wedge pressure is not different for patients with chronic heart failure who are limited by either dyspnea or by fatigue (Sullivan 1989).

The excess ventilation apparently compensates for the abnormal pulmonary hemodynamics in order to maintain normal blood gas tensions (Metra et al. 1992). Patients who are limited in exercise by particularly severe dyspnea rather than fatigue, generally have a lower $\dot{V}O_2$ peak, indicative of more advanced left ventricular dysfunction (Andreas et al. 1995). Some patients with left ventricular dysfunction rely on more rapid, shallow breathing during exercise than do healthy individuals (Yokoyama et al. 1994; see figure 3.39). Many heart failure patients demonstrate an increase in physiological dead space ventilation (Myers et al. 1992).

Wada and associates (1992) measured pulmonary blood flow with radioisotopically labeled albumin and documented an abnormal distribution of pulmonary blood flow in some heart failure patients (see figure 3.40). Patients with severe heart failure ($\dot{V}O_2$ peak < 12-14 ml/kg/min) may demonstrate an

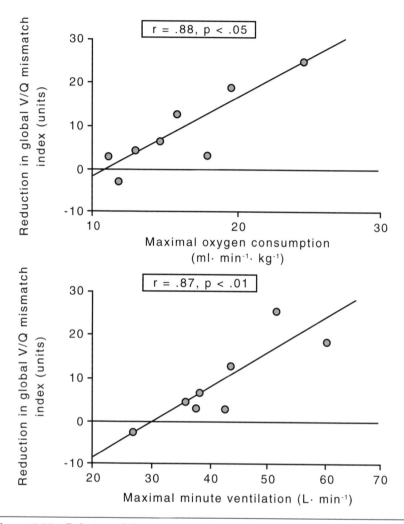

Figure 3.35 Relation of the reduction in global ventilation-perfusion (V/Q) mismatch index with maximal oxygen consumption and maximal minute ventilation.

Reprinted, with permission, from Uren NG, Davies SW, Agnew JE, Irwin AG, Jordan SI, Hilson AJW, Lipkin DP. Reduction of mismatch of global ventilation and perfusion on exercise is related to exercise capacity in chronic heart failure. *Br Heart J* 70:241-246. Copyright 1993 BMJ Publishing Group.

oscillating pattern of increasing and decreasing minute ventilation (see figure 3.41). This phenomenon is most apparent during the transition from rest to light intensity exercise and is dampened with heavy exercise (Kremser et al. 1987). Yajima and coworkers (1994) simultaneously measured $\dot{V}_E$ and LVEF during exercise and found complimentary oscillations in both variables in

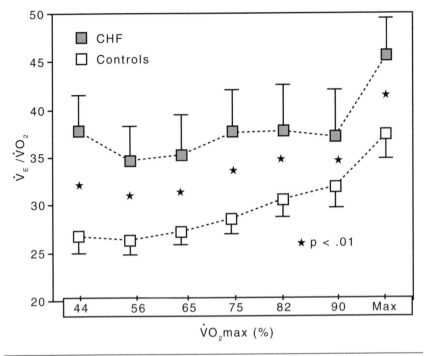

Figure 3.36 Changes in ventilatory equivalent for oxygen ($\dot{V}_E/\dot{V}O_2$) expressed as a percentage of $\dot{V}O_2$ max for patients with chronic heart failure (CHF) and normal controls (mean ± 2 SEM).

Reprinted, with permission, from Myers J, Salleh A, Buchanan N, Smith D, Neutel J, Bowes E, Froelicher VF. 1992. Ventilatory mechanisms of exercise intolerance in chronic heart failure. *Am Heart J* 124:710-719.

patients with severe heart failure; they postulate the abnormal oscillating breathing pattern is a result of changes in pulmonary blood flow.

Patients with chronic left ventricular dysfunction are usually limited in graded exercise by either dyspnea or general fatigue. Clark and associates (1995) investigated the potential mechanisms of limiting symptoms in a population of 222 patients with chronic heart failure. Table 3.8 provides selected variables for patients with either limiting fatigue or dyspnea. As can be seen, etiology of left ventricular dysfunction, $\dot{V}O_2$peak, ventilatory equivalents, echocardiographic variables, and serum electrolytes were similar for both groups of patients. These authors concluded that fatigue and dyspnea, in chronic heart failure, are apparently due to the same underlying physiologic abnormalities.

In summary, patients with chronic heart failure commonly exhibit the following pulmonary characteristics:

- Mild pulmonary function abnormalities

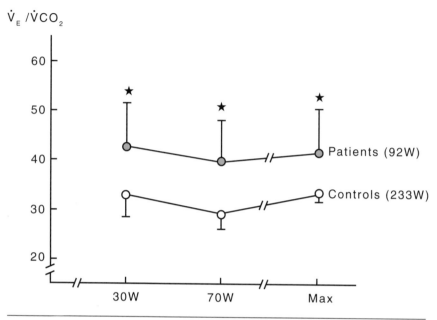

Figure 3.37   Ventilatory equivalent for carbon dioxide ($\dot{V}_E/\dot{V}CO_2$) during cycle exercise in chronic heart failure (n = 13) and healthy subjects (n = 8). The mean peak cycle exercise intensity in watts (w) is indicated for both groups. ★ p < .05.

Reprinted, with permission, from Sovijarvi ARA, Naveri H, Leinonen H. Ineffective ventilation during exercise in patients with chronic congestive heart failure. *Clin Phys* 12:403. Copyright 1992 Blackwell Science Ltd.

- Normal arterial blood gases and arterial saturation at rest and during exercise in compensated heart failure
- Excessive ventilation during exercise as evidenced by elevated ventilatory equivalents for O_2 and CO_2
- Limiting symptom of dyspnea in many patients during exercise

Graded Exercise Testing in Chronic Heart Failure

Formal exercise testing is helpful in the evaluation, treatment, and rehabilitation of patients with left ventricular dysfunction. Common reasons for graded exercise testing in this patient population include the following:

- Accurate determination of exercise capacity, amount of disability, and symptom severity
- Prognosis assessment and potential listing for cardiac transplantation

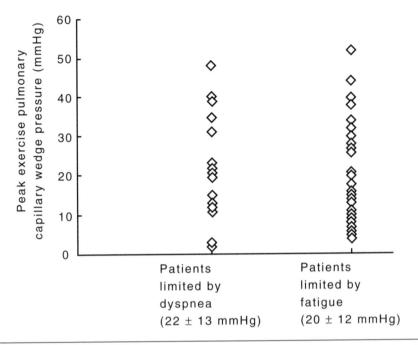

Figure 3.38 Peak cycle exercise pulmonary capillary wedge pressure in heart failure patients limited by dyspnea (n = 16) or fatigue (n = 44).

From Sullivan MJ. 1989. Exercise intolerance in CHF: Role of peripheral factors. *Cardio* April:137-144. Reproduced with permission of S. Karger AG, Basel.

- Exercise prescription
- Determination of the effects of treatment such as medications, surgery, exercise training, weight reduction
- Assessment of myocardial ischemia

Myocardial ischemia may be assessed in patients with coronary artery disease by several methods, as discussed earlier in this chapter. The direct measurement of oxygen uptake and related variables is extremely useful and provides more objective data regarding aerobic capacity than does using estimates of $\dot{V}O_2$ from the exercise test peak workload. The ventilatory anaerobic threshold may be obtained in most patients and may be useful in exercise prescription. In my experience, combining imaging techniques for determination of myocardial ischemia (nuclear or echo) with concurrent gas analysis is feasible and worthwhile for selected patients with coronary atherosclerosis.

The following sections provide basic information regarding exercise testing for patients with chronic heart failure. Excellent comprehensive

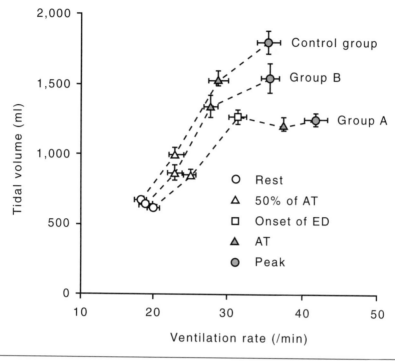

Figure 3.39   The average tidal volume-ventilation rate in heart failure and normal subjects divided into two subgroups based on the presence (A) or absence (B) of exertional dyspnea (ED). The data represent four reference time points: rest, 50% of the anaerobic threshold (AT), at the AT, and at peak exercise. For group A, an additional time point of ED onset is included.

Reprinted, with permission, from Yokoyama H, Sato H, Hori M, Takeda H, Kamada T. 1994. A characteristic change in ventilation made during exertional dyspnea in patients with chronic heart failure. *Chest* 106:1007-1013.

information concerning cardiopulmonary exercise testing is contained in the texts by Wasserman and associates (1994), Wasserman (1996) and Myers (1996).

Pretest Patient Evaluation

A recent examination by a qualified physician is a requirement, and may include the following components:

- Cardiovascular examination
- Electrocardiogram
- Blood analyses (especially serum potassium for patients taking diuretics; hemoglobin concentration)

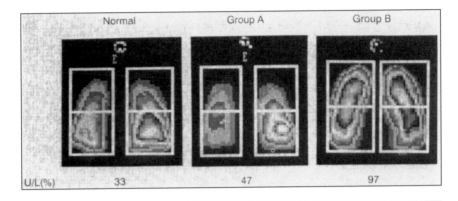

Figure 3.40 Pulmonary perfusion scintigrams representative of three groups (normal control, Group A = chronic heart failure patients with normal exercise ventilation, Group B = chronic heart failure patients with excessive exercise ventilation). U/L = ratio of upper to lower counts. The pulmonary blood flow is distributed more to the upper lung in Group B patients.

Reprinted, with permission, from Wada O, Asanoi H, Miyagi K, Ishizaka S, Kameyama T, Seto H, Sasayama S. 1992. Importance of abnormal lung perfusion in excessive exercise ventilation in chronic heart failure. *Am Heart J* 125:790-798.

- Medication use
- Exercise habits and symptoms
- Musculoskeletal status
- Measure of left ventricular function (LVEF)
- Spirometry, if determination of cause of dyspnea is of prime concern

Contraindications for exercise testing, specifically for patients with heart failure, include uncompensated heart failure, the presence of rales, uncontrolled edema; uncontrolled arrhythmias; Class IV symptoms; unstable angina; or hypokalemia.

Exercise Testing Equipment

Standard equipment found in most laboratories includes a 12-lead electrocardiograph, blood pressure cuff and stethoscope, exercise devices, emergency equipment including defibrillator, gas exchange measurement system, and pulse oximeter.

The most commonly used exercise devices are the motorized treadmill and cycle ergometer. For patients with lower extremity limitations to exercise, a combination arm-leg ergometer or an arm ergometer may be useful. Patients with pulmonary hypertension or significant other pulmonary disease should have arterial oxygen saturation continuously monitored during exercise. Commercially available metabolic measurement carts are reliable and quite accurate in the measurement of pulmonary gas

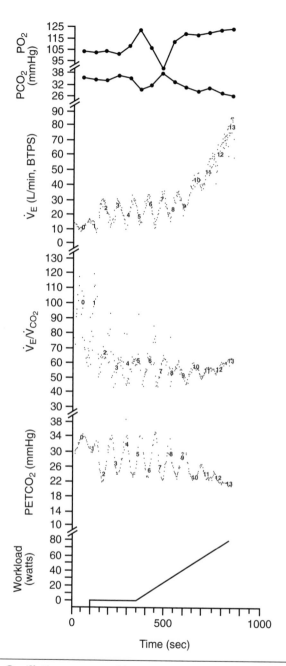

Figure 3.41 Oscillating pattern of increasing and decreasing minute ventilation (V_E) and associated variables (V_E/VCO_2 = ventilatory equivalent for carbon dioxide; PETCO$_2$ = end-tidal carbon dioxide partial pressure) during incremental cycle exercise in a patient with chronic heart failure.

Reprinted from *The American Journal of Cardiology*, 59, Kremser CB, O'Toole MF, Leff AR., Oscillatory hyperventilation in severe congestive heart failure secondary to idiopathic dilated cardiomyopathy or to ischemic cardiomyopathy, 903, Copyright 1987, with permission from Excerpta Medica Inc.

Table 3.8 Comparison of Heart Failure Patients Whose Symptoms at Peak Exercise Were Dyspnea or Fatigue

	Fatigue (n = 62)	Dyspnea (n = 160)
$\dot{V}O_2$peak (ml/kg/min)	15.7 ± 5.6	15.1 ± 4.6
Exercise duration (sec)	603 ± 545	513 ± 458
$\dot{V}_E/\dot{V}CO_2$	2.6 ± 1.3	3.0 ± 1.2
LVEF (%)	24.9 ± 11.8	22.0 ± 12.2
LVEDP (mmHg)	15.4 ± 8.7	18.9 ± 10.0

None of the comparisons were significantly different.
$\dot{V}_E/\dot{V}CO_2$ = ventilatory equivalent for carbon dioxide; LVEF = left ventricular ejection fraction; LVEDP = left ventricular end-diastolic pressure.

From *Eur Heart J*, 16, Clark AL, Sparrow JL, Coats AJS. Muscle fatigue and dyspnea in chronic heart failure: Two sides of the same coin? 49-52, 1995, by permission of the publisher W B Saunders Company Limited London.

exchange, as long as calibration and routine maintenance schedules are followed.

Exercise Test Protocols and Procedures

Protocols for exercise testing of patients with chronic heart failure are designed to start at metabolic requirements of approximately 2 METs, and increase in intensity by 1-2 METs each stage. These protocols are often more conservative in initial exercise intensity and rate of progression of intensity than protocols generally used in cardiology. Stage duration is generally 1-2 minutes, although ramp protocols with continuously increasing work rates may be used. Table 3.9 shows the treadmill protocol used in my laboratory. The vast majority of patients can perform well with this protocol that begins at 2 mph, 0% grade, and increases in work intensity by 1-2 METs each 2 minutes. For patients who cannot walk 2 mph, we commonly modify the Naughton protocol with a treadmill speed of 1-1.5 mph. Cycle protocols may begin at 0 external work intensity and increase in work rate by 5-20 watts each minute, depending upon the size of the patient. A description of ramp protocols is provided in the Wasserman and colleagues text (1994).

The electrocardiogram should be continuously observed and blood pressure measured before exercise begins and during each exercise stage, as well as at least once during the recovery phase. Expired air is analyzed continuously for one minute before exercise, during exercise, and for at least one minute after peak exercise. Modern metabolic measurement carts display gas exchange variables continuously in a real-time format. Symp-

Table 3.9   Mayo Clinic Cardiopulmonary Treadmill Exercise Testing Protocol

Stage	Speed (mph)	Grade (%)	Duration (min)
1	2.0	0	2
2	2.0	7.0	2
3	2.0	14.0	2
4	3.0	12.5	2
5	3.0	17.5	2
6	3.4	18.0	2
7	3.8	20.0	2
8	5.0	18.0	2
9	5.5	20.0	2
10	6.0	22.0	2
11	6.5	24.0	2

toms are assessed by having patients use hand signals or "point at" charts (patients cannot speak during gas exchange measurement). The Borg perceived scale is useful in understanding the patient-perceived level of effort. The test endpoints are as follows:

- Symptom limitation, usually fatigue or dyspnea, but moderate to severe angina is also an endpoint
- Hypotension; systolic blood pressure during exercise below rest blood pressure
- Sustained ventricular arrhythmias
- Sustained supraventricular arrhythmias
- ST segment evidence of severe myocardial ischemia
- Patient request to discontinue exercise

Patients are encouraged to exercise to the point of limiting fatigue or dyspnea, unless another termination criterion is met. In my laboratory, an active recovery phase of three minutes of walking at 1.7 mph, 0% grade occurs after peak exercise. This is followed by three minutes of sitting rest.

Exercise Test Personnel

In my practice, a physician is available in the immediate testing area during exercise testing. The testing is carried out by either an experienced exercise physiologist, nurse, or exercise specialist with the assistance of an exercise technologist. An ACLS certified person is always available. For properly screened chronic heart failure patients, exercise testing is remarkably safe (Tristani et al. 1987).

Test Interpretation

The electrocardiogram, blood pressure, and symptoms are interpreted as for other clinical populations. Arterial desaturation is present if $SaO_2\%$ decreases by more than 4% during exercise. Gas exchange variables require a trained eye for interpretation. In my institution, exercise physiologists with the PhD degree are responsible for test interpretation. The rate of rise in $\dot{V}O_2$, $\dot{V}O_2$peak, and the presence of a plateau in $\dot{V}O_2$ are all important variables in the interpretation. I prefer to use the term $\dot{V}O_2$peak for the highest measured $\dot{V}O_2$ during graded exercise tests rather than $\dot{V}O_2$max in clinical populations such as CHF patients. Pulmonary ventilation during peak exercise and the ventilatory equivalents are also scrutinized carefully. The ventilatory anaerobic threshold is determined. Case examples appear in chapter 5.

For patients with myocardial ischemia or chronic heart failure, exercise responses may be abnormal, as reviewed in this chapter. Graded exercise testing of these high-risk patients provides useful information from diagnostic, prognostic, treatment, and rehabilitation perspectives.

References

Ambrosio G, Betocchi S, Pace L, Losi MA, Perrone-Filardi P, Soricelli A, Piscione F, Taube J, Squame F, Salvatore M, Weiss JL, Chiariello M. 1996. Prolonged impairment of regional contractile function after resolution of exercise-induced angina: Evidence of myocardial stunning in patients with coronary artery disease. *Circulation* 94:2455-2464.

American College of Sports Medicine. 1995. *Guidelines for Exercise Testing and Exercise Prescription*. 5th ed. Philadelphia: Lea & Febiger.

Andreas S, Vonhof S, Kreuzer H, Figulla HR. 1995. Ventilation and dyspnea during exercise in patients with heart failure. *Eur Heart J* 16:1886-1891.

Arnold JMO, Ribeiro JP, Colucci WS. 1990. Muscle blood flow during forearm exercise in patients with severe heart failure. *Circulation* 82:465-472.

Buller NP, Jones D, Poole-Wilson PA. 1991. Direct measurement of skeletal muscle fatigue in patients with chronic heart failure. *Br Heart J* 65:20-24.

Buller NP, Poole-Wilson PA. 1990. Mechanism of the increased ventilatory response to exercise in patients with chronic heart failure. *Br Heart J* 63:281-283.

Carter CL, Amundsen LR. 1977. Infarct size and exercise capacity after myocardial infarction. *J Appl Physiol* 42:782-785.

Clark AL, Coats AJS. 1994. Usefulness of arterial blood gas estimations during exercise in patients with chronic heart failure. *Br Heart J* 71:528-530.

Clark AL, Sparrow JL, Coats AJS. 1995. Muscle fatigue and dyspnea in chronic heart failure: Two sides of the same coin? *Eur Heart J* 16:49-52.

Cohen-Solal A, Aupetit JF, Gueret P, Kolsky H, Zannad F. 1994. Can anaerobic threshold be used as an end-point for therapeutic trials in heart failure? Lessons from a multicentre randomized placebo-controlled trial. *Eur Heart J* 15:236-241.

Cohen-Solal A, Aupetit JF, Page E, Geneves M, Gourgon R. 1996. Transient fall in oxygen intake during exercise in congestive heart failure. *Chest* 110:841-844.

Cohen-Solal A, Chabernaud JM, Gourgon R. 1990. Comparison of oxygen uptake during bicycle exercise in patients with chronic heart failure and in normal subjects. *J Am Coll Cardiol* 16:80-85.

Cohen-Solal A, Gourgon R. 1991. Assessment of exercise tolerance in chronic congestive heart failure. *Am J Cardiol* 67:36C-40C.

Cohen-Solal A, Laperche T, Morvan D, Geneves M, Caviezel B, Gourgon R. 1995. Prolonged kinetics of recovery of oxygen consumption after maximal graded exercise in patients with chronic heart failure: Analysis with gas exchange measurements and NMR spectroscopy. *Circulation* 91:2924-2932.

Cohen-Solal A, Zannad F, Kayanakis JG, Gueret P, Aupetit JF, Kolsky H. 1991. Multicentre study of the determination of peak oxygen uptake and ventilatory threshold during bicycle exercise in chronic heart failure: Comparison of graphical methods, interobserver variability and influence of the exercise protocol. *Eur Heart J* 12:1055-1063.

Colucci WS, Riberio JP, Rocco MB, Quigg RJ, Creager MA, Marsh JD, Gauthier DF, Hartley LF. 1989. Impaired chronotropic response to exercise in patients with congestive heart failure: Role of postsynaptic β-adrenergic desensitization. *Circulation* 80:314-323.

Cross AM, Higginbotham MB. 1995. Oxygen deficit during exercise testing in heart failure: Relation to submaximal exercise tolerance. *Chest* 107:904-908.

Dahan M, Aubry N, Baleynaud S, Ferreira B, Yu J, Gourgon R. 1995. Influence of preload reserve on stroke volume response to exercise in patients with left ventricular systolic dysfunction: A Doppler echocardiographic study. *J Am Coll Cardiol* 25:680-686.

Daida H, Allison TG, Johnson BD, Squires RW, Gau GT. 1996. Further increase in oxygen uptake during early active recovery following maximal exercise in chronic heart failure. *Chest* 109:47-51.

Davies SW, Emery TM, Watling ML, Wannamethee G, Lipkin DP. 1991. A critical threshold of exercise capacity in the ventilatory response to exercise in heart failure. *Br Heart J* 65:179-183.

Ellestad MH. 1996. *Stress Testing: Principles and Practice*. 4th ed. Philadelphia: F.A. Davis Co.

Hashimoto M, Okamoto M, Yamagata T, Yamane T, Watanabe M, Tsuchioka Y, Matsuura H, Kajiyama G. 1993. Abnormal systolic blood pressure response during exercise recovery in patients with angina pectoris. *J Am Coll Cardiol* 22:659-664.

Hayashida W, Kumada T, Kohno F, Noda M, Ishikawa N, Kambayashi M, Kawai C. 1993. Post-exercise oxygen uptake kinetics in patients with left ventricular dysfunction. *Int J Cardiol* 38:63-72.

Hecht HS, Karahalios SE, Ormiston JA, Schnugg SJ, Hopkins JM, Singh BN. 1982. Patterns of exercise response in patients with severe left ventricular dysfunction: Radionuclide ejection fraction and hemodynamic cardiac performance evaluations. *Am Heart J* 104:718-724.

Hess OM, Buchi M, Kirkeeide R, Niederer P, Anliker M, Gould KL, Krayenbuhl HP. 1990. Potential role of coronary vasoconstriction in ischaemic heart disease: Effect of exercise. *Eur Heart J* (II Suppl B):58-64.

Hossack KF. 1987. Cardiovascular responses to dynamic exercise. *Cardiol Clin* 5:147-156.

Hurst JW. 1992. Coronary heart disease: The overview of the clinician. In *Rehabilitation of the Coronary Patient*. 3rd ed. Wenger NK, Hellerstein HK (eds). New York: Churchill Livingstone, pp. 3-18.

Iskandrian AS, Kegel JG, Lemlek J, Heo J, Cave V, Iskandrian B. 1992. Mechanism of exercise-induced hypotension in coronary artery disease. *Am J Cardiol* 69:1517-1520.

Janicki JS, Gupta S, Ferris ST, McElroy PA. 1990. Long-term reproducibility of respiratory gas exchange measurements during exercise in patients with stable cardiac failure. *Chest* 97:12-17.

Jondeau G, Katz SD, Toussaint JF, Dubourg O, Monrad ES, Bourdarias JP, LeJemtel TH. 1993. Regional specificity of peak hyperemic response in patients with congestive heart failure: Correlation with peak aerobic capacity. *J Am Coll Cardiol* 22:1399-1402.

Katz SD, Berkowitz R, LeJemtel TH. 1992. Anaerobic threshold detection in patients with congestive heart failure. *Am J Cardiol* 69:1565-1569.

Katz SD, Krum H, Khan T, Knecht M. 1996. Exercise-induced vasodilation in forearm circulation of normal subjects and patients with congestive heart failure: Role of endothelium-derived nitric oxide. *J Am Coll Cardiol* 28:585-590.

Kemp GJ, Thompson CH, Stratton JR, Brunotte F, Conway M,

Adamopoulos S, Arnolda L, Radda GK, Rajagopalan B. 1996. Abnormalities in exercising skeletal muscle in congestive heart failure can be explained in terms of decreased mitochondrial ATP synthesis, reduced metabolic efficiency, and increased glycogenolysis. *Heart* 76:35-41.

Keteyian SJ, Marks CRC, Brawner CA, Levine AB, Kataoka T, Levine TB. 1996. Responses to arm exercise in patients with compensated heart failure. *J Cardiopulm Rehabil* 16:366-371.

Kitzman DW, Brubaker P, Stewart KP, Miller HS, Ettinger WH. 1997. Aerobic capacity in elderly patients with heart failure due to primary diastolic dysfunction is severely reduced and is similar to systolic dysfunction. *J Am Coll Cardiol* 29:464A.

Kitzman DW, Higginbotham MB, Cobb FR, Sheikh KH, Sullivan MJ. 1991. Exercise intolerance in patients with heart failure and preserved left ventricular function: Failure of the Frank-Starling mechanism. *J Am Coll Cardiol* 17:1065-1072.

Koike A, Hiroe M, Adachi H, Yajima T, Yamauchi Y, Nogami A, Ito H, Miyahara Y, Korenaga M, Marumo F. 1994. Oxygen uptake kinetics are determined by cardiac function at onset of exercise rather than peak exercise in patients with prior myocardial infarction. *Circulation* 90:2324-2332.

Koike A, Yajima T, Adachi H, Shimizu N, Kano H, Sugimoto K, Niwa A, Marumo F, Hiroe M. 1995. Evaluation of exercise capacity using submaximal exercise at a constant work rate in patients with cardiovascular disease. *Circulation* 91:1719-1724.

Kraemer MD, Kubo SH, Rector TS, Brunsvold N, Bank AJ. 1993. Pulmonary and peripheral vascular factors are important determinants of peak oxygen uptake in patients with heart failure. *J Am Coll Cardiol* 21:641-648.

Kremser CB, O'Toole MF, Leff AR. 1987. Oscillatory hyperventilation in severe congestive heart failure secondary to idiopathic dilated cardiomyopathy or to ischemic cardiomyopathy. *Am J Cardiol* 59:900-905.

LeJemtel TH, Laing C, Stewart DK, Kirlin PC, McIntyre KM, Robertson TH, Moore A, Cahill L, Galvao M, Wellington KL, Garces C, Held P. 1994. Reduced peak aerobic capacity in asymptomatic left ventricular systolic dysfunction: A substudy of the studies of left ventricular dysfunction (SOLVD). *Circulation* 90:2757-2760.

Liang C, Stewart DK, LeJemtel TH, Kirlin PC, McIntyre KM, Robertson T, Brown R, Moore AW, Wellington KL, Cahill L, Galvao M, Woods PA, Garces C, Held P. 1992. Characteristics of peak aerobic capacity in symptomatic and asymptomatic subjects with left ventricular dysfunction. *Am J Cardiol* 69:1207-1211.

Magnusson G, Isberg B, Karlberg KE, Sylven C. 1994. Skeletal muscle strength and endurance in chronic congestive heart failure secondary to idiopathic dilated cardiomyopathy. *Am J Cardiol* 73:307-309.

Mancini D, Donchez L, Levine S. 1997. Acute unloading of the work of breathing extends exercise duration in patients with heart failure. *J Am Coll Cardiol* 29:590-596.

Marie PY, Escanye JM, Brunotte F, Robin B, Walker P, Zannad F, Robert J, Gilgenkrantz JM. 1990. Skeletal muscle metabolism in the leg during exercise in patients with congestive heart failure. *Clin Sci* 78:515-519.

Massie BM, Conway M, Rajagopalan B, Yonge R, Frostick S, Ledingham J, Sleight P, Radda G. 1988. Skeletal muscle metabolism during exercise under ischemic conditions in congestive heart failure, evidence for abnormalities unrelated to blood flow. *Circulation* 78:320-326.

Massie B, Conway M, Yonge R, Frostick S, Ledingham J, Sleight P, Radda G, Rajagopalan B. 1987. Skeletal muscle metabolism in patients with congestive heart failure: Relation to clinical severity and blood flow. *Circulation* 76:1009-1019.

Mayo Clinic Cardiovascular Working Group on Stress Testing. 1996. Cardiovascular stress testing: A description of the various types of stress tests and indications for their use. *Mayo Clin Proc* 71:43-52.

McParland C, Krishnan B, Wang Y, Gallagher CG. 1992. Inspiratory muscle weakness and dyspnea in chronic heart failure. *Am Rev Respir Dis* 146:467-472.

Messner-Pellenc P, Brasileiro C, Ahmaidi S, Mercier J, Ximenes C, Grolleau R, Prefaut C. 1995. Exercise intolerance in patients with chronic heart failure: Role of pulmonary diffusing limitations. *Eur Heart J* 16:201-209.

Metra M, DeiCas L, Panina G, Visioli O. 1992. Exercise hyperventilation chronic congestive heart failure, and its relation to functional capacity and hemodynamics. *Am J Cardiol* 70:622-628.

Metra M, Raddino R, DeiCas L, Visioli O. 1990. Assessment of peak oxygen consumption, lactate and ventilatory thresholds and correlation with resting and exercise hemodynamic data in chronic congestive heart failure. *Am J Cardiol* 65:1127-1133.

Milani RV, Mehra MR, Reddy TK, Lavie CJ, Ventura HO. 1996. Ventilation/carbon dioxide production ratio in early exercise predicts poor functional capacity in congestive heart failure. *Heart* 76:393-396.

Miller TD, Gibbons RJ, Squires RW, Allison TG, Gau GT. 1993. Sinus node deceleration during exercise as a marker of significant narrowing of the right coronary artery. *Am J Cardiol* 71:371-373.

Minotti JR, Christoph I, Oka R, Weiner MW, Wells L, Massie BM. 1991. Impaired skeletal muscle function in patients with congestive heart failure: Relationship to systemic exercise performance. *J Clin Invest* 88:2077-2082.

Minotti JR, Pillay P, Oka R, Wells L, Christoph I, Massie BM. 1993. Skeletal muscle size: Relationship to muscle function in heart failure. *J Appl Physiol* 75:373-381.

Muller AF, Batin P, Evans S, Hawkins M, Cowley AJ. 1992. Regional blood flow in chronic heart failure: The reason for lack of correlation between patients' exercise tolerance and cardiac output. *Br Heart J* 67:478-481.

Myers J, Salleh A, Buchanan N, Smith D, Neutel J, Bowes E, Froelicher VF. 1992. Ventilatory mechanisms of exercise intolerance in chronic heart failure. *Am Heart J* 124:710-719.

Myers JN. 1996. *Essentials of Cardiopulmonary Exercise Testing.* Champaign, IL: Human Kinetics.

Paraskevaidis IA, Kremastinos DT, Kassimatis AS, Karavolias GK, Kordosis GD, Kyriakides ZS, Toutouzas PK. 1993. Increased response of diastolic blood pressure to exercise in patients with coronary artery disease: An index of latent ventricular dysfunction? *Br Heart J* 69:507-511.

Pouleur H, Hanet C, Rousseau MF, VanEyll C. 1990. Relation of diastolic function and exercise capacity in ischemic left ventricular dysfunction: Role of β-agonists and β-antagonists. *Circulation* 82(Suppl I):89-96.

Predel HG, Knigge H, Prinz U, Kramer HJ, Stalleicken D, Rost RE. 1995. Exercise increases endothelin-1 plasma concentrations in patients with coronary artery disease: Modulatory role of LDL cholesterol and of pentaerithrityltetranitrate. *J Cardiovasc Pharm* 26(Suppl 3):497-501.

Reading JL, Goodman JM, Plyley MJ, Floras JS, Liu PP, McLaughlin PR, Shephard RJ. 1993. Vascular conductance and aerobic power in sedentary and active subjects and heart failure patients. *J Appl Physiol* 74:567-573.

Riley M, Bell N, Elborn JS, Stanford CF, Buchanan KD, Nicholls NP. 1993. Metabolic responses to graded exercise in chronic heart failure. *Eur Heart J* 14:1484-1488.

Riley M, Elborn JS, Bell N, Stanford CF, Nicholls DP. 1990. Substrate utilization during exercise in chronic cardiac failure. *Clin Sci* 79:89-95.

Riley M, Porszasz J, Stanford CF, Nicholls DP. 1994. Gas exchange responses to constant work rate exercise in chronic heart failure. *Br Heart J* 72:150-155.

Roubin GS, Anderson SD, Shen WF, Choong CY, Alwyn M, Hillery S, Harris PJ, Kelly DT. 1990. Hemodynamic and metabolic basis of impaired exercise tolerance in patients with severe left ventricular dysfunction. *J Am Coll Cardiol* 15:986-994.

Rundquist B, Eisenhofer G, Elan M, Friberg P. 1997. Attenuated cardiac sympathetic responsiveness during dynamic exercise in patients with heart failure. *Circulation* 95:940-945.

Sietsema KE, Ben-Dor I, Zhang YY, Sullivan C, Wasserman K. 1994. Dynamics of oxygen uptake for submaximal exercise and recovery in patients with chronic heart failure. *Chest* 105:1693-1700.

Smith RF, Johnson G, Ziesche S, Bhat G, Blankenship K, Cohn JN. 1993. Functional capacity in heart failure: Comparison of methods for assessment and their relation to other indexes of heart failure. *Circulation* 87(Suppl VI):88-93.

Sovijarvi ARA, Naveri H, Leinonen H. 1992. Ineffective ventilation during exercise in patients with chronic congestive heart failure. *Clin Physiol* 12:399-408.

Squires RW, Williams WL. 1993. Coronary atherosclerosis and myocardial infarction. In *American College of Sports Medicine Resource Manual for Guidelines for Exercise Testing and Prescription.* 2nd ed. Philadelphia: Lea & Febiger, pp.168-186.

Stenberg J, Astrand PO, Ekblom B, Royce J, Saltin B. 1967. Hemodynamic response to work with different muscle groups, sitting and supine. *J Appl Physiol* 22:61-70.

Sullivan MJ. 1989. Exercise intolerance in CHF: Role of peripheral factors. *Cardiol* April:137-144.

Sullivan MJ, Green HJ, Cobb FR. 1991. Altered skeletal muscle metabolic response to exercise in chronic heart failure: Relation to skeletal muscle aerobic enzyme activity. *Circulation* 84:1597-1607.

Sullivan MJ, Knight JD, Higginbotham MB, Cobb FR. 1989. Relation between central and peripheral hemodynamics during exercise in patients with chronic heart failure: Muscle blood flow is reduced with maintenance of arterial perfusion pressure. *Circulation* 80:769-781.

Tomai F, Ciavolella M, Cren F, Gaspardone A, Versaci F, Giannitti C, Scali D, Chiariello L, Gioffre PA. 1993. Left ventricular volumes during exercise in normal subjects and patients with dilated cardiomyopathy assessed by first-pass radionuclide angiography. *Am J Cardiol* 72:1167-1171.

Tristani FE, Hughes CV, Archibald DG, Sheldhl LM, Cohn JN, Fletcher R. 1987. Safety of graded symptom-limited exercise testing in patients with congestive heart failure. *Circulation* 76(Suppl VI):54-58.

Uren NG, Davies SW, Agnew JE, Irwin AG, Jordan SI, Hilson AJW, Lipkin DP. 1993a. Reduction of mismatch of global ventilation and perfusion on exercise is related to exercise capacity in chronic heart failure. *Br Heart J* 70:241-246.

Uren NG, Davies SW, Jordan SL, Lipkin DP. 1993b. Inhaled bronchodilators increase maximum oxygen consumption in chronic left ventricular failure. *Eur Heart J* 14:744-750.

Volterrani M, Clark AL, Ludman PF, Swan JW, Adamopoulos S, Piepoli M, Coats AJS. 1994. Predictors of exercise capacity in chronic heart failure. *Eur Heart J* 15:801-809.

Wada O, Asanoi H, Miyagi K, Ishizaka S, Kameyama T, Seto H, Sasayama S. 1992. Importance of abnormal lung perfusion in excessive exercise ventilation in chronic heart failure. *Am Heart J* 125:790-798.

Wasserman K (ed). 1996. *Exercise Gas Exchange in Heart Disease*. Armonk, NY: Future Publishing Co.

Wasserman K, Hansen JE, Sue DY, Whipp BJ, Casaburi R. 1994. *Principles of Exercise Testing and Interpretation*. 2nd ed. Philadelphia: Lea & Febiger.

Weber KT, Janicki JS, McElroy PA, Reddy HK. 1988. Monitoring physical activity in ambulatory patients with chronic heart failure. *Cardiovasc Clin* 18:141-154.

Wilson JR, Martin JL, Ferraro N. 1984a. Impaired skeletal muscle nutritive flow during exercise in patients with congestive heart failure: Role of cardiac pump dysfunction as determined by the effect of dobutamine. *Am J Cardiol* 53:1308-1315.

Wilson JR, Martin JL, Schwartz D, Ferraro N. 1984b. Exercise intolerance in patients with chronic heart failure: Role of impaired nutritive flow to skeletal muscle. *Circulation* 69:1079-1087.

Wilson JR, Rayos G, Yeoh TK, Gothard P. 1995. Dissociation between peak exercise oxygen consumption and hemodynamic dysfunction in potential heart transplant candidates. *J Am Coll Cardiol* 26:429-435.

Yajima T, Koike A, Sugimoto K, Miyahara Y, Marumo F, Hiroe M. 1994. Mechanism of periodic breathing in patients with cardiovascular disease. *Chest* 106:142-146.

Yamani MH, Sahgal P, Wells L, Massie BM. 1995. Exercise intolerance in chronic heart failure is not associated with impaired recovery of muscle function or submaximal exercise performance. *J Am Coll Cardiol* 25:1232-1238.

Yokoyama H, Sato H, Hori M, Takeda H, Kamada T. 1994. A characteristic change in ventilation made during exertional dyspnea in patients with chronic heart failure. *Chest* 106:1007-1013.

Zhang YY, Wasserman K, Sietsema KE, Ben-Dov I, Barstow TJ, Mizumoto G, Sullivan CS. 1993. Oxygen uptake kinetics in response to exercise: A measure of tissue anaerobiosis in heart failure. *Chest* 103:735-741.

CHAPTER 4

Benefits of Exercise Training for High-Risk Cardiac Patients

This chapter reviews the results of various investigations of exercise training for patients with myocardial ischemia or chronic heart failure. It emphasizes potential benefits of training.

Exercise Training in Patients With Myocardial Ischemia

In general, exercise training improves the exercise capacity of patients with coronary artery disease. However, coronary patients are a heterogeneous group and do not always demonstrate a predictable and consistent response to exercise training. Patients may differ in respect to the extent of atherosclerotic disease, the amount and severity of myocardial ischemia, and in systolic and diastolic left ventricular function.

Several investigators (Clausen and Trap-Jensen 1970; Redwood et al. 1972) have reported increases in $\dot{V}O_2$max of 10% to 30% or more in typical coronary patients after training. The rate of improvement is greatest during the first three months of training, but further increases in aerobic capacity may occur for six months or more (Foster et al. 1984). As shown in figure 4.1, similar improvements in $\dot{V}O_2$max have been documented for patients after

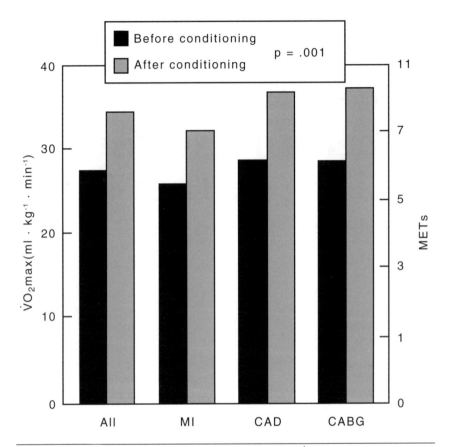

Figure 4.1 Increase in maximal oxygen uptake ($\dot{V}O_2$max) resulting from exercise training in patients with myocardial infarction (MI), coronary artery bypass surgery (CABG), and angiographically documented coronary artery disease (CAD). All = all coronary patients; METs = multiples of resting metabolic rate.

Reprinted, with permission, from Hartung GH, Rangel R. 1981. Exercise training in post-myocardial infarction patients: Comparison of results with high risk coronary and post-bypass patients. *Archives of Physical Medicine and Rehabilitation* 62:147-150.

myocardial infarction, coronary bypass surgery, and for patients with angiographically demonstrated disease without a cardiac event (Hartung and Rangel 1981). However, patients with documented ischemia that occurs during exercise training generally do not exhibit as much improvement in aerobic capacity as do coronary patients without ischemia (Arvan 1988; Ades et al. 1989).

Researchers have investigated exercise programs for coronary patients employing a lower than customary intensity of exercise with the goals of enhancing compliance with exercise training and minimizing the risks of habitual exercise. Two investigations compared the benefits obtained from high- and low-intensity exercise programs. The results demonstrated similar gains in aerobic capacity from programs using an intensity of < 45% of VO_2max or a target heart rate of 20 beats per minute above the resting heart rate while standing and from the more traditional programs (60% to 70% of VO_2max) (Blumenthal et al. 1988; Gobel et al. 1991).

Some coronary patients do not improve maximal exercise capacity as a result of training, but do improve submaximal exercise performance (endurance). Such improvements include a lower heart rate and VO_2 for a given absolute submaximal exercise intensity and greatly prolonged endurance times at a standard exercise pace (Ades et al. 1993).

Peripheral Versus Central Circulatory Adaptation

The improvement in aerobic capacity after exercise training in patients with coronary artery disease has historically been assumed to be due to peripheral tissue adaptations leading to an increased a-$\overline{v}O_2$ difference (increased oxygen extraction from arterial blood) rather than an increase in maximal cardiac output. Mitochondrial oxidative enzyme activity and the rate of regeneration of phosphocreatine have been shown to improve in coronary patients as a result of training (Ferguson et al. 1982; Adamopoulos et al. 1993). Whether exercise cardiac output increases as a result of training has been controversial.

Some researchers from the 1970s, during the early years of the investigation of the effects of exercise training in coronary artery disease, reported an increase in exercise cardiac output after training in some cardiac patients (Clausen and Trap-Jensen 1970; Paterson et al. 1979). Investigators at Washington University in St. Louis, Missouri, sought to address the issue of central circulatory adaptation to exercise training in coronary patients. They maximized the training stimulus by gradually increasing the training intensity and duration over the course of one year for highly motivated patients, some with demonstrable exercise-induced ischemia. The final training program of their studies consisted of 60 minutes of exercise, five days per week, at an intensity of 70% to 90% of VO_2max (Hagberg 1991). Mean VO_2max increased by approximately 40%. Evidence for an improvement in exercise cardiac output was indicated by the following findings: echocardiographic evidence of improved left ventricular myocardial fractional shortening and mean velocity of shortening (Ehsani et al. 1982), an average 18% increase in stroke volume measured during submaximal exercise (35% to 65% of VO_2max) (see figure 4.2) (Hagberg et al. 1983), improvement in systolic time intervals (Martin et al. 1984), increased exercise left ventricular ejection fraction (Ehsani et al. 1986), and reversal of observed exercise-related drop in systolic blood pressure (Martin and Ehsani 1987).

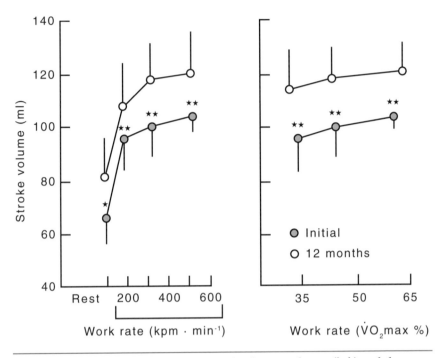

Figure 4.2   Stroke volume at the same absolute work rate (left) and the same relative work rate (right) before and after 12 months of intense exercise training in patients with coronary artery disease. VO₂max = maximal oxygen uptake. ★ p < .05. ★★ p < .01.

Reproduced, with permission, from Hagberg JM, Ehsani AA, Holloszy JO. Effect of 12 months of intense exercise training on stroke volume in patients with coronary artery disease. *Circulation* 67:1197. Copyright 1983 American Heart Association.

In summary, exercise training in patients with coronary artery disease and exercise-induced myocardial ischemia usually results in an improvement in $\dot{V}O_2$peak and submaximal exercise endurance. The improvements are the result of beneficial changes in peripheral circulatory function and perhaps of an increase in exercise cardiac output in some patients.

Improvement in Exercise-Related Myocardial Ischemia

Exercise training may improve exercise-induced myocardial ischemia. There is evidence that exercise reduces the myocardial oxygen demand and improves oxygen delivery to the heart muscle. As seen in figure 4.3, after training, for a standard submaximal exercise intensity, the rate-pressure product (systolic blood pressure × heart rate, an index of myocardial oxygen requirement) is reduced. This enables the patient to perform a higher intensity of physical activity before exceeding the ischemic threshold

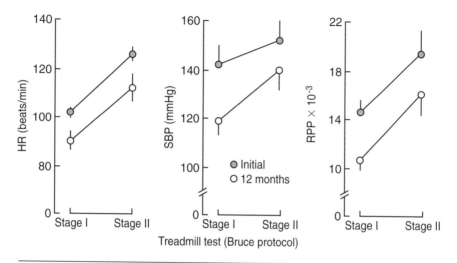

Figure 4.3   Effects of 12 months of exercise training on heart rate (HR), systolic blood pressure (SBP), and the rate-pressure product (RPP) at stages I and II of the Bruce treadmill testing protocol. All variables were significantly lower (p < .01) after training.

Reprinted from *The American Journal of Cardiology*, 50, Ehsani AA, Martin WH, Heath GW, Coyle EF., Cardiac effects of prolonged and intense exercise training in patients with coronary artery disease, 249, Copyright 1982, with permission from Excerpta Medica Inc.

(the rate-pressure product that corresponds to the onset of measurable myocardial ischemia).

Some investigators have reported that the rate-pressure product at the ischemic threshold is increased by habitual exercise, independent of changes in blood lipids or anti-ischemic medications, suggesting that myocardial blood flow may have improved (Raffo et al. 1980; Laslett et al. 1985). Reductions in exercise-induced ischemia, measured by exercise thallium perfusion scanning, of 54% and 34% have been reported (Schuler et al. 1988; Todd et al. 1991). The reduction in ischemia at peak exercise in these studies was not the result of a lower maximal rate-pressure product. Decreased blood viscosity is a potential mechanism for the reduction in ischemia. Some investigators believe that enhanced coronary collateral flow may be another reason for the improvement, although no direct evidence for enhancement of collateral vessels with exercise training exists (Franklin 1991; Kennedy et al. 1976).

Exercise Training and the Progression of Coronary Atherosclerosis

Exercise training in sufficient amounts appears to slow the progression of, or even reverse, coronary atherosclerosis. German investigators examined the effects of one year of supervised, moderate intensity exercise training on the angiographic appearance of coronary lesions (Hambrecht et al. 1993). Approximately 60 coronary patients were randomized to control conditions or exercise training. Both groups were instructed in a low-fat, low-cholesterol diet and were given information regarding the benefits of regular aerobic exercise. The exercise group performed a home exercise program and the controls were left to the usual care of their primary physicians. No blood lipid-improving medications were used in either group. Angiographically determined progression of coronary atherosclerosis occurred in 45% of controls and 10% of exercise subjects. Some degree of regression of lesions was observed in 28% of exercisers versus 6% of controls. Figure 4.4 shows that partial regression of atherosclerosis was seen only in patients who expended an average of 2,200 or more kilocalories per week in physical activity (approximately 5-6 hours of moderate intensity exercise per week).

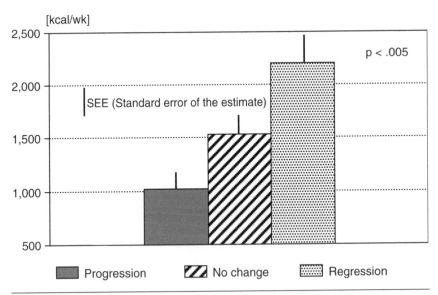

Figure 4.4   Energy expenditure (kcal/wk) in patients with coronary atherosclerosis and changes in atherosclerotic lesion morphology over one year. The highest levels of exercise energy expenditures were observed in patients showing regression of disease.

Reprinted from *Journal of the American College of Cardiology*, 22, Hambrecht R, Niebauer J, Marburger C, Grunze M, Kalberer B, Hauer K, Schlierf G, Kubler W, Schuler G., Various intensities of leisure time physical activity in patients with coronary artery disease: Effects on cardiorespiratory fitness and progression of coronary atherosclerotic lesions, 471, Copyright 1993, with permission from the American College of Cardiology.

Summary of Exercise Training Benefits in Myocardial Ischemia

As discussed in the foregoing section, beneficial increases and improvements in the following variables have been reported in the investigations:

- $\dot{V}O_2$peak
- Submaximal exercise endurance
- Maximal cardiac output
- Maximal stroke volume
- Skeletal muscle mitochondrial oxidative enzyme activity
- Phosphocreatine resynthesis
- Exercise left ventricular ejection fraction
- Coronary atherosclerosis regression
- Ischemic threshold

A decrease has been reported for the following variables (a beneficial effect):

- Exercise rate-pressure product
- Myocardial oxygen requirement at rest and during submaximal exercise
- Severity and extent of exercise-related myocardial ischemia
- Exercise hypotension
- Coronary atherosclerosis progression

Exercise Training for Patients With Chronic Heart Failure

Until relatively recently, exercise training was not considered part of the standard treatment program for patients with severe left ventricular dysfunction. Rest from physical activity was considered an important component of the time-honored treatment, given the fact that for a time, patients with congestive symptoms require rest, as well as diuresis and optimization of digoxin and vasodilator therapy in order to improve symptomatically. However, even for patients who appear well compensated, physicians have been reluctant to recommend or allow exercise training for the following additional concerns:

- Exercise may increase cardiac filling pressures and hasten the eventual progression of ventricular dysfunction and clinical deterioration

- Exercise may induce myocardial ischemia in patients with ischemic cardiomyopathy
- Exercise may potentiate life-threatening ventricular arrhythmias
- Patients may not benefit from training

Patients with signs of uncompensated heart failure such as rales, uncontrolled edema, ventricular tachycardia at rest, and class four symptoms (unable to walk one block) are candidates for more aggressive medical and surgical therapy, not exercise training. However, limiting physical activity in patients with compensated heart failure may not only be unnecessary, but detrimental since it may worsen disability (deconditioning effect of inactivity). Although disuse and deconditioning are not the only causes of poor physical work capacity in patients with chronic heart failure, they play a crucial role in initiating adverse metabolic changes in skeletal muscle that can only be reversed by physical training (Coats et al. 1992). Fortuitously, investigators in the late 1970s and mid 1980s began the systematic study of exercise training for chronic heart failure patients as an extension of the cardiac rehabilitation programs of the era.

Early Studies of the Safety and Efficacy of Exercise Training in Patients With Left Ventricular Dysfunction

The first investigation of exercise training in patients with low left ventricular ejection fractions was reported by Letac and colleagues in 1977. As part of a larger exercise training program for patients with coronary artery disease, the authors performed a subgroup analysis on eight patients with LVEFs of < 45%. The patients exercised (walk, jog, cycle, row) for eight weeks, three sessions per week, at a heart rate of 80% of maximum determined by symptom-limited cycle exercise testing. After training, these patients exhibited a slightly lower heart rate (-10 beats/min) at a standard submaximal exercise work intensity, a small increase in maximal exercise capacity (+5 watts). No changes, either positive or negative, in LVEF, left ventricular end-diastolic volume, or other echocardiographic indices of systolic function were found.

Lee and associates, in 1979, published results of a trial of exercise training in 18 men with coronary artery disease and LVEFs of < 40% (mean 35%, range 27% to 40%). Exercise training occurred three to five times per week (walk, cycle, jog), at an intensity of 70% to 85% of maximal heart rate for an average of 19 months (range 12-42 months). Treadmill exercise time (Bruce protocol) improved by an average of approximately one minute. Thirteen of the 18 patients improved exercise duration. Left heart catheterizations were performed before and after the period of exercise training and no changes were found in the following variables: pulmonary artery pressure, left ventricular end-diastolic pressure and volume, cardiac and stroke volume index (at rest), and LVEF. One death occurred but was apparently not related to the exercise training.

In 1982, Conn et al. reported results from an approximately one-year (range 4-37 months) exercise training program for nine men and one woman with coronary artery disease and LVEFs of approximately 20% (range 13% to 26%). Exercise consisted of walking, cycling, and jogging for 45 minutes, three to five times per week at 70% to 80% of maximal heart rate. Estimated maximum METs increased by an average of 1.5 with seven of the 10 patients demonstrating an improvement in exercise duration. There were no exercise-related adverse events although two deaths occurred during the study.

Squires and coworkers, in 1987, reported the rehabilitation outcome in 18 men and two women with ischemic heart disease and LVEFs of < 25% (mean 21%, range 14% to 25%). Eighteen of the patients had a history of an anterior wall myocardial infarction. Eleven had experienced ventricular tachycardia, eleven had congestive symptoms during hospitalization, and one patient had chronic atrial fibrillation. Sixteen of the patients began the rehabilitation program within three weeks of their myocardial infarction. The exercise program was supervised for the first eight weeks and consisted of cycle ergometry and treadmill walking at an intensity of 50% to 60% of capacity with a gradual increase in duration to 30-40 minutes per session with a frequency of three sessions per week. Upon completion of the eight-week supervised program, patients were encouraged to continue exercise training and risk factor modification steps such as avoidance of tobacco and a low-fat, low-cholesterol diet. One patient entered a community-based exercise program and the others elected to perform home exercise training.

Questionnaires asking about employment status, exercise habits, and patient perceptions of disability were mailed an average of 19 months after graduation from the supervised exercise program (range 13-35 months). Patient medical records were reviewed for survival data approximately 30 months postprogram. Three hundred and twelve supervised exercise sessions were performed by the subjects without any serious medical emergencies. Mean treadmill exercise test time improved by approximately 38% by the end of the supervised exercise program.

After the 30-month follow-up interval, four patients had died (deaths occurred at 6, 13, 15, and 19 months), yielding an annualized mortality of approximately 8%. All deaths were cardiac. Three were sudden and there was no temporal association with exercise training. One death resulted from biventricular failure.

All 16 survivors had been fully employed prior to their most recent cardiac event: 14 with sedentary occupations and two with moderately active jobs. At the time of the patient questionnaire, nine of 16 (56%) were working full-time, including the two patients with more active job responsibilities. Two of the patients who died had also returned to full-time work before their deaths. One patient was retired (age 73 years), but was fully active. Six patients were medically disabled from their heart disease. Thirty-one percent of patients reported the ability to perform all desired activities (no subjective impairment). Slight to moderate impairment was reported by 46% and severe impairment by 23%. The vast majority (92%) reported participation in at least one formal exercise training session per week with the following modes of activity: walking, cycling, jogging, and swimming. The authors concluded that these patients had experienced a generally favorable rehabilitation outcome and that patients with poor left ventricular function should not be categorically excluded from cardiac rehabilitation programs.

Thus, these early investigations of exercise training in patients with chronic heart failure demonstrated the safety and potential benefits of such programs. All of these studies were limited by a lack of a nonexercising control group and the possibility of selection bias (the patients in these studies may not be representative of the typical patient with severe left ventricular dysfunction). In the late 1980s and early 1990s, several important investigations provided a more scientific basis for the recommendation of exercise training in the setting of left ventricular dysfunction.

Landmark Investigations of the Effects of Exercise Training in Chronic Heart Failure

Sullivan et al. published results from an elegant experiment of exercise training in chronic heart failure patients in 1988 and 1989. They extensively studied 16 patients (mean LVEF 24%, range 9% to 33%), nine with coronary artery disease and seven with idiopathic dilated cardiomyopathy, before and after a four- to six-month training program. Patients exercised an average of four hours per week (range 2.4-5.0 hours per week) at an intensity of 75% of $\dot{V}O_2$max using a combination of cycling, walking, jogging, and stair climbing. Cycle $\dot{V}O_2$max was measured monthly and exercise intensity was adjusted accordingly. Four patients did not complete the study (one sudden cardiac death unrelated to the training program, one orthopedic injury, two patients with progressive congestive failure symptoms). The following cycle ergometer symptom-limited graded exercise tests were performed before and after the training program with extensive patient instrumentation:

1. Swan-Ganz catheters in the right pulmonary artery and femoral vein, cannula in the left brachial artery (for the determination of right atrial, pulmonary artery, and systemic arterial pressures; arterial oxygen saturation and content; peripheral venous and mixed venous oxygen content; arterial and venous lactate concentration)
2. Expired air analysis

3. Multiple gated equilibrium radionuclide angiogram during each work stage
4. Thermistor determined leg blood flow
5. Direct Fick determined cardiac output
6. Left ventricular end-diastolic and end-systolic volume calculated from the stroke volume and LVEF

Results for maximal exercise from the initial and final exercise tests are provided in table 4.1. The $\dot{V}O_2$peak increased by an average of 23% (17-21 ml/kg/min), primarily as a result of a widening of the a-$\bar{v}O_2$ difference. Maximal heart rate and respiratory exchange ratio were unchanged. Single leg blood flow increased by approximately 0.5 L/min. The increase in $\dot{V}O_2$max was present by day 75 of training (see figure 4.5), with a further improvement in aerobic capacity up to day 165 (end of the study).

Table 4.1   Selected Variables at Peak Exercise for 12 Chronic Heart Failure Patients Before and After 4 to 6 Months of Exercise Training

	Before	After	p value
$\dot{V}O_2$peak (L/min)	1.11 ± 0.33	1.40 ± 0.40	< .01
(ml/kg/min)	16.8 ± 3.7	20.6 ± 4.7	< .01
Heart rate (beats/min)	145 ± 14	146 ± 14	NS
Respiratory exchange ratio	1.32 ± 0.14	1.36 ± 0.15	NS
Arterial lactate (mmol/L)	6.7 ± 2.0	7.6 ± 2.7	NS
Work intensity (kpm/min)	520 ± 105	613 ± 119	< .01
Cardiac output (L/min)	8.9 ± 2.9	9.9 ± 3.2	.13
a-$\bar{v}O_2$ diff (ml/dl)	13.1 ± 1.4	14.6 ± 2.3	<.05
Single leg blood flow (L/min)	2.5 ± 0.7	3.0 ± 0.8	<.01

a-$\bar{v}O_2$ diff = arterial-mixed venous oxygen differences.

Reprinted, with permission, from Sullivan MJ, Higginbotham MB, Cobb FR. Exercise training in patients with severe left ventricular dysfunction: Hemodynamic and metabolic effects. *Circulation* 78:506-515.

As shown in figure 4.6, there was a trend for stroke volume and cardiac output to increase with training. Since leg blood flow was higher after training and cardiac output was only marginally improved, the ability of the leg skeletal muscle to vasodilate apparently increased with training. This is consistent with the hypothesis of Sinoway (1988), that some of the impaired

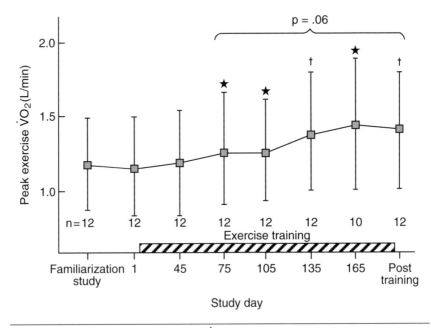

Figure 4.5   Time course of change in $\dot{V}O_2$peak with exercise training in patients with chronic heart failure. ★ $p < .05$, † $p < .01$ vs. day 1.

Reproduced, with permission, from Sullivan MJ, Higginbotham MB, Cobb FR. Exercise training in patients with severe left ventricular dysfunction: Hemodynamic and metabolic effects. *Circulation* 78:511. Copyright 1988 American Heart Association.

vasodilatory response observed in chronic heart failure is a result of deconditioning. Submaximal exercise $\dot{V}O_2$ was not altered by training but submaximal heart rate for each exercise stage was approximately 10 beats/min lower after training. There were no changes observed in mean arterial pressure, pulmonary capillary wedge pressure, right atrial pressure, and mean pulmonary artery pressure (see figure 4.7).

As can be seen in figure 4.8, left ventricular ejection fraction, and end-systolic and end-diastolic volumes at rest and during each exercise stage were not affected by the training. A small, but statistically significant, increase in arterial oxygen content (without a change in arterial oxygen saturation) was found. Symptomatically, the patients improved their New York Heart Association class from a mean of 2.4-1.3.

Ventilatory variables during the incremental cycle exercise tests before and after exercise training are shown in figure 4.9. For a given submaximal work intensity and for maximal exercise, minute ventilation, carbon dioxide production, and the respiratory exchange ratio were lower after training. There was no change found for the ventilatory equivalent for carbon dioxide. The ventilatory anaerobic threshold increased by 2 ml/kg/min (see figure 4.10).

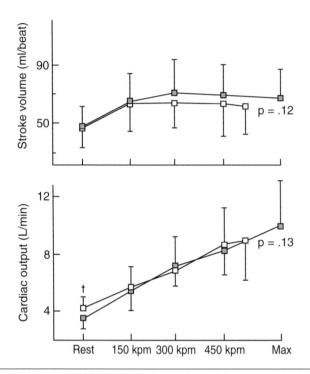

Figure 4.6   Rest and exercise stroke volume and cardiac output before (□) and after (■) exercise training in patients with chronic heart failure. † p < .01. (The x-axis represents cycle workload [kpm/min].)

Reproduced, with permission, from Sullivan MJ, Higginbotham MB, Cobb FR. Exercise training in patients with severe left ventricular dysfunction: Hemodynamic and metabolic effects. *Circulation* 78:509-510. Copyright 1988 American Heart Association.

In addition to the graded cycle ergometer exercise tests, patients also performed a constant submaximal exercise intensity (approximately 79% of pretraining $\dot{V}O_2$max) cycle endurance test with continuous expired air analysis. Exercise time for the constant work test increased significantly from 938 ± 410 to 1,429 ± 691 seconds. Figure 4.11 shows that after training the heart rate, minute ventilation, ventilatory equivalent for carbon dioxide, and respiratory exchange ratio all declined significantly. Thus, the investigators demonstrated a substantial training effect, largely as a result of peripheral adaptations including an increase in peak leg blood flow. No evidence for adverse cardiac effects was found and the patients were symptomatically improved as a result of training. Responses to submaximal exercise, including the ventilatory anaerobic threshold, heart rate, and minute ventilation were also improved after training. The magnitude of the improvements in exercise tolerance was similar to that observed in other cardiac patients with well-preserved left ventricular function.

A second groundbreaking investigation was published by Coats and

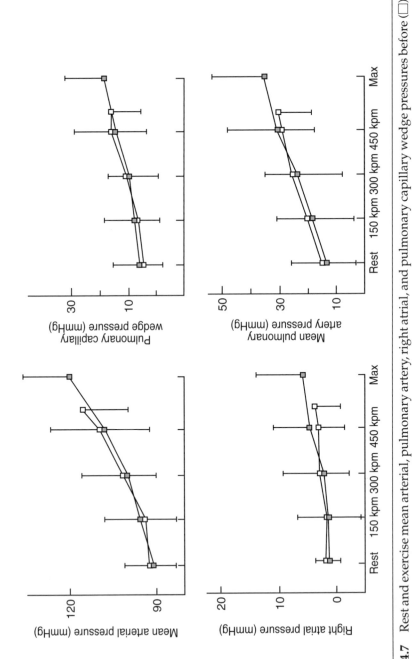

Figure 4.7 Rest and exercise mean arterial, pulmonary artery, right atrial, and pulmonary capillary wedge pressures before (□) and after (■) exercise training in patients with chronic heart failure.

Reproduced, with permission, from Sullivan MJ, Higginbotham MB, Cobb FR. Exercise training in patients with severe left ventricular dysfunction: Hemodynamic and metabolic effects. *Circulation* 78:509. Copyright 1988 American Heart Association.

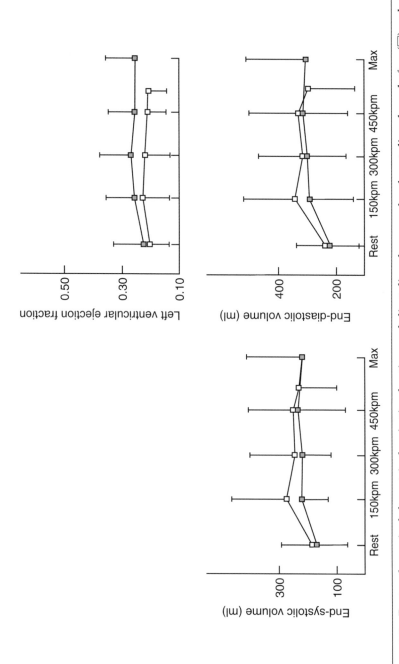

Figure 4.8 Rest and exercise left ventricular ejection fraction, end-diastolic volume, and end-systolic volume before (□) and after (■) exercise training in patients with chronic heart failure.

Reproduced, with permission, from Sullivan MJ, Higginbotham MB, Cobb FR. Exercise training in patients with severe left ventricular dysfunction: Hemodynamic and metabolic effects. *Circulation* 78:510. Copyright 1988 American Heart Association.

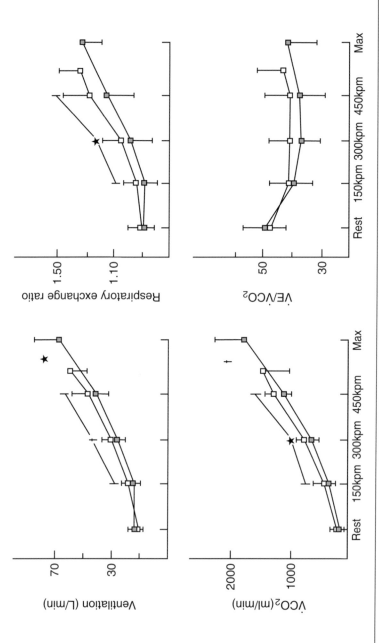

Figure 4.9 Rest and exercise ventilation, respiratory exchange ratio, carbon dioxide production ($\dot{V}CO_2$), and the ventilatory equivalent for carbon dioxide ($\dot{V}_E/\dot{V}CO_2$) before (□) and after (■) exercise training in patients with chronic heart failure. ★ $p < .05$; † $p < .01$.

Reproduced, with permission, from Sullivan MJ, Higginbotham MB, Cobb FR. Exercise training in patients with chronic heart failure delays ventilatory anaerobic threshold and improves submaximal exercise performance. *Circulation* 79:326. Copyright 1989 American Heart Association.

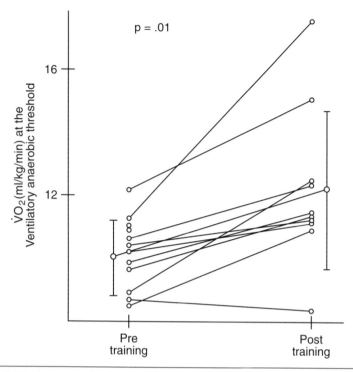

Figure 4.10   Changes in the ventilatory anaerobic threshold with exercise training in 12 patients with chronic heart failure.

Reproduced, with permission, from Sullivan MJ, Higginbotham MB, Cobb FR. Exercise training in patients with chronic heart failure delays ventilatory anaerobic threshold and improves submaximal exercise performance. *Circulation* 79:327. Copyright 1989 American Heart Association.

associates as a preliminary report in 1990, and as a completed study in 1992. These authors sought to determine the magnitude of the training effect in terms of both the cardiovascular and autonomic nervous systems. Importantly, the study was a randomized, crossover design of eight weeks' duration. Half of the 19 subjects were randomized to begin either exercise or no exercise (normal activity) at the beginning of the study and after eight weeks crossed over to the other group. All of the subjects had ischemic left ventricular dysfunction with a mean LVEF of 20%, and none was limited by angina pectoris. Two subjects did not complete the study (one death due to progressive congestive failure, one cardiac transplantation). Of the remaining 17 subjects, 12 had suffered an anterior wall myocardial infarction and 15 took angiotensin-converting enzyme inhibiting drugs.

The subjects performed cycle ergometer exercise training at their homes, five days per week, 20 minutes duration, at a heart rate of 60% to 80% of maximum. Compliance with the exercise program was monitored by an

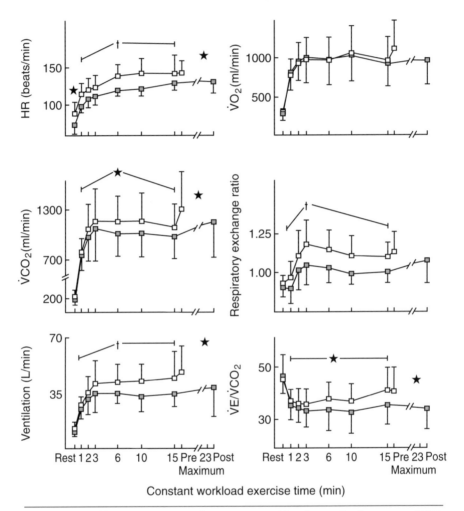

Figure 4.11   Changes in rest and constant workload exercise heart rate (HR), oxygen uptake ($\dot{V}O_2$), carbon dioxide production ($\dot{V}CO_2$), respiratory exchange ratio, ventilation, and the ventilatory equivalent for carbon dioxide ($\dot{V}_E/\dot{V}CO_2$) before (□) and after (■) exercise training in patients with chronic heart failure. ★ p < .05, † p < .01.

Reproduced, with permission, from Sullivan MJ, Higginbotham MB, Cobb FR. Exercise training in patients with chronic heart failure delays ventilatory anaerobic threshold and improves submaximal exercise performance. *Circulation* 79:327. Copyright 1989 American Heart Association.

rpm measuring device installed on each cycle. The control group (no exercise) was instructed to avoid all above normal physical activity. Graded cycle ergometer exercise tests with analysis of expired air were performed at each eight-week interval together with 24-hour Holter monitoring for the determination of heart rate variability as an index of autonomic nervous system function. Power spectral analysis of the R to R wave variability was performed, including both a high frequency component as an index of parasympathetic activity and a low frequency component as an index of sympathetic activity. Blood norepinephrine kinetics were measured and patient symptoms scored on a standard scale. Stroke volume was estimated by pulsed-Doppler echocardiographic assessment of the ascending aortic blood flow velocity during a separate cycle exercise test in the supine posture specifically for this purpose.

During the study, there were no exercise-related adverse side effects and compliance with home exercise was good (77%). No changes in body weight or medications occurred. The $\dot{V}O_2$max increased by an average of 18% (13-16 ml/kg/min) and maximal heart rate remained unchanged. There was a tendency for the slope of minute ventilation to carbon dioxide production to decrease (see figure 4.12) consistent with a reduction in excess ventilation

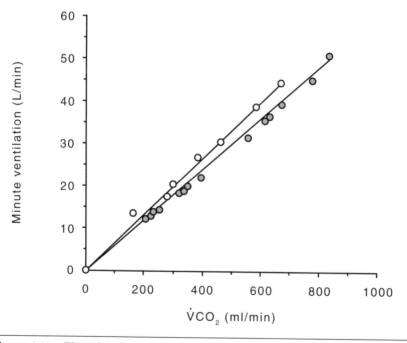

Figure 4.12   The relationship of minute ventilation to carbon dioxide production ($\dot{V}CO_2$) in a single chronic heart failure patient before (○) and after (●) exercise training.

Reproduced, with permission, from Coats AJS, Adamopoulos S, Radaelli A, McCance A, Meyer TE, Bernardi L, Solda PL, Davey P, Ormerod O, Forfar C, Conway J, Sleight P. Controlled trial of physical training in chronic heart failure: Exercise performance, hemodynamics, ventilation, and autonomic function. *Circulation* 85:2123. Copyright 1992 American Heart Association.

during exercise. Figure 4.13 shows that cardiac output, estimated by echocardiography, improved at both submaximal and maximal exercise intensities (6.3-7.1 L/min at maximal exercise) after training.

Spectral analysis results for low frequency (sympathetic activity) and high frequency (parasympathetic activity) domains are given in figure 4.14. The observed reduction in percentage low frequency and the increase in percentage high frequency after exercise training is consistent with a shift from more sympathetic activity to more parasympathetic activity. Whole body norepinephrine spillover was also reduced after training (381 versus 321 ng/min/m²). These data are consistent with a reduction in neurohormonal activation as a result of habitual physical activity.

Symptoms of breathlessness and fatigue were improved after training and patients reported an increase in daily spontaneous physical activity. The study demonstrated the feasibility and safety of home exercise training for patients with chronic heart failure. In addition to the benefit of an improved aerobic capacity, patients also demonstrated improvement for an

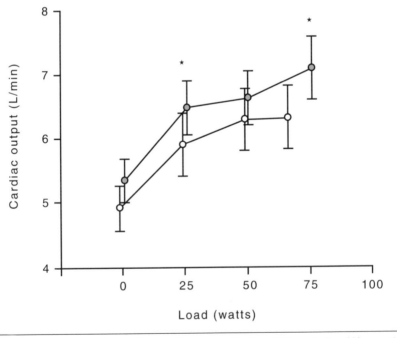

Figure 4.13   Rest and exercise cardiac output before (○) and after (◉) exercise training in patients with chronic heart failure. ★ p < .05.

Reproduced, with permission, from Coats AJS, Adamopoulos S, Radaelli A, McCance A, Meyer TE, Bernardi L, Solda PL, Davey P, Ormerod O, Forfar C, Conway J, Sleight P. Controlled trial of physical training in chronic heart failure: Exercise performance, hemodynamics, ventilation, and autonomic function. *Circulation* 85:2124. Copyright 1992 American Heart Association.

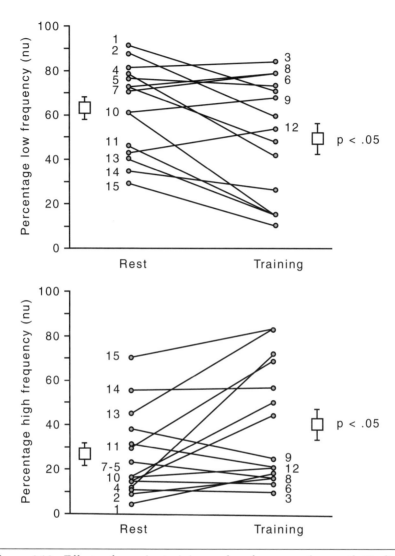

Figure 4.14   Effects of exercise training on low frequency (sympathetic division of the autonomic nervous system) and high frequency (parasympathetic division of the autonomic nervous system) spectral analysis in patients with chronic heart failure. nu = normalized units.

Reproduced, with permission, from Coats AJS, Adamopoulos S, Radaelli A, McCance A, Meyer TE, Bernardi L, Solda PL, Davey P, Ormerod O, Forfar C, Conway J, Sleight P. Controlled trial of physical training in chronic heart failure: Exercise performance, hemodynamics, ventilation, and autonomic function. *Circulation* 85:2126. Copyright 1992 American Heart Association.

index of cardiac output as well as for autonomic nervous system function. The patients were carefully selected, however, and none had limiting angina or significant ventricular arrhythmias.

A second randomized, controlled trial of exercise training in patients with left ventricular dysfunction was reported in 1991 by Jette and colleagues (1991). The trial took place at a German rehabilitation hospital and included 15 patients with LVEFs of < 30% and large anterior wall myocardial infarctions occurring less than 10 weeks before onset of the trial. Randomization to exercise or control treatments resulted in similar baseline characteristics of the groups. Exercise training was performed on a daily basis for only four weeks and included walking, cycling, jogging, calisthenics, and relaxation activities for a total duration of up to 2.5 hours interspersed during the day. No changes in echocardiographic variables were observed (neither positive nor negative changes). In the control patients, no improvement in aerobic capacity occurred, but VO_2max did increase in exercising patients by approximately 200 ml/min. This study indicated that an aggressive exercise training program begun early after myocardial infarction complicated by severe left ventricular dysfunction results in a substantial training effect in selected patients.

The final landmark investigation was published by Hambrecht et al. (1995a, 1995b). Twenty-two patients with either idiopathic dilated cardiomyopathy or ischemic left ventricular dysfunction (mean LVEF 27%) were randomly assigned to exercise training or control groups.

The six-month training program consisted of a high volume of exercise including 40 minutes of daily cycle ergometry at 70% of VO_2max at the patients' homes, and two supervised group exercise sessions per week consisting of 60 minutes of games, calisthenics, and walking. Cycle ergometer graded exercise tests were performed before and after the six-month study period. Expired air analysis was performed during exercise testing in addition to hemodynamic measurements using femoral vein and pulmonary artery Swan-Ganz catheters. Percutaneous needle biopsies of the vastus lateralis for skeletal muscle metabolic profiling was also performed.

No exercise-related incidents occurred. One patient died from cardiac arrest. Table 4.2 provides oxygen transport system data before and after training. As can be seen, heart rate at rest declined while maximal heart rate increased as a result of exercise training. Cardiac output also increased significantly (+2.2 L/min). Maximal oxygen uptake and the ventilatory anaerobic threshold increased substantially. Plasma lactate concentration during submaximal exercise improved in the exercise but not in the control group. Cytochrome C oxidase activity, a marker for skeletal muscle aerobic metabolic capacity, improved by an average of 41%. Plasma norepinephrine concentration decreased at rest and during submaximal exercise in the training group. These authors recently reported that their exercising subjects experienced a partial "reshift" from type II (fast twitch) to type I (slow twitch) muscle fibers of the vastus lateralis (Hambrecht et al. 1997).

For six of the subjects who were considered at the highest risk and were awaiting cardiac transplantation (mean LVEF 16%), VO_2peak did increase

Table 4.2   Oxygen Transport System Variables for 22 Patients With Chronic Heart Failure Before and After 6 Months of Exercise Training

	Baseline	6-Months	Change
Rest heart rate (beats/min)	88 ± 18	82 ± 18*	-6 ± 12
Peak exercise heart rate (beats/min)	163 ± 27	174 ± 22*	11 ± 13
Peak exercise cardiac output (L/min)	11.9 ± 4.0	14.1 ± 3.3*	2.2 ± 2.5
Anaerobic threshold (L/min)	0.9 ± 0.2	1.1 ± 0.2*	0.2 ± 0.2
$\dot{V}O_2$peak (ml/kg/min)	17.5 ± 5.1	23.3 ± 4.2*	5.8 ± 3.6

* $p < .05$.

Reprinted from *Journal of the American College of Cardiology*, 25, Hambrecht R, Neibauer J, Fiehn E, Kalberer B, Offner B, Hauer K, Riede U, Schlierf G, Kubler W, Schuler G., Physical training in patients with stable chronic heart failure: Effects on cardiorespiratory fitness and ultrastructural abnormalities of leg muscle, 1242, Copyright 1995, with permission from the American College of Cardiology.

with training from 1.07 ± 0.30 to 1.27 ± 0.21 L/min. Functional class improved from approximately 3.0-2.3.

After two years of continued exercise training in these patients, no change in LVEF was seen, but end-diastolic diameter did decrease from approximately 70-66 mm. Aerobic capacity increased further to 1.6 L/min. These authors concluded that a duration of six months was adequate for most of the training adaptations to occur and that the effects persist for at least two years without risk of worsening heart failure as a result of exercise training.

After a period of exercise training with an improvement in exercise capacity, activity restriction (detraining) results in a loss of the improvement in fitness in patients with CHF (Meyer et al. 1997b). Maintenance of training benefits requires life-long exercise participation.

Additional Studies of Exercise Training in Chronic Heart Failure

Several other investigators have made important contributions to our understanding of the responses and benefits of training in patients with left ventricular dysfunction. Adamopoulos et al. (1995) included a large (n = 70) group of patients with a mean LVEF of 23% in an extension of the investigation of Coats and associates (1992). These patients were apparently not highly selected and included essentially all comers who did not have a contraindication for exercise.

A randomized crossover design using home cycle ergometry demonstrated a modest increase in directly measured $\dot{V}O_2$peak (+1.6 ml/kg/min) and a reduction in resting plasma norepinephrine concentration (-30 pg/ml). In order to determine if a baseline variable predicts improvement in exercise capacity, multiple regression analysis was performed with etiology of heart failure, age, medications, body surface area, LVEF, plasma norepinephrine concentration, sympathovagal balance, symptomatic status, and history of coronary bypass surgery as dependent variables. None of these factors was a significant predictor of change in exercise capacity after training.

Two randomized, controlled trials of approximately six months of exercise training provided some new insights. Keteyian and colleagues (1996) demonstrated a 16% improvement in VO_2peak and approximately a 10 beat/min increase in maximal heart rate with three 45-minute exercise sessions per week at an intensity of 60% to 80% of the heart rate reserve. In a similar study, Kiilavuori and associates (1996) reported only a trend for improved aerobic capacity, but a substantial increase in submaximal exercise endurance (47% improvement in exercise time at 85% of baseline VO_2peak).

Dubach and colleagues (1997a, 1997b) performed a two-month randomized, controlled trial of high volume exercise training in 25 men with ischemic left ventricular dysfunction. Exercising patients walked two hours each day plus performed four weekly cycle ergometer sessions of 40 minutes at 70% to 80% of heart rate reserve. VO_2peak increased by an average of 29% as a result of an increase in directly measured cardiac output (12.0 ± 1.8 L/min to 13.7 ± 2.5 L/min) and arteriovenous oxygen difference. Magnetic resonance imaging before and after the period of exercise training revealed no adverse effects on left ventricular volume, ejection fraction or wall thickness.

Several investigations have increased our knowledge of the changes that occur in skeletal muscle of chronic heart failure patients with habitual exercise. Skeletal muscle biopsies of the anterolateral thigh were performed by Belardinelli et al. (1995b) before and after an eight-week cycle exercise program in 27 patients with either ischemic or idiopathic dilated cardiomyopathy (18 patients in the exercise treatment group, nine patients were nonrandomized controls; mean LVEF 30%). Graded exercise testing with hemodynamic monitoring demonstrated a 17% increase in VO_2peak, no changes in ventricular volumes or indices of left ventricular function (echocardiographic measurements), and no change in exercise stroke volume or cardiac output. Table 4.3 shows that skeletal muscle adaptations occurred only in the training group, including an increase in fiber size, and in volume density of mitochondria. These data are consistent with the concept that the majority of the increase in aerobic capacity resulting from exercise training in heart failure in short-term programs is likely due to enhanced oxidative capacity of skeletal muscle.

Some investigators have used ^{31}P magnetic resonance spectroscopy to

Table 4.3   Skeletal Muscle Biopsy Results With 8 Weeks of Exercise Training in Patients With Chronic Left Ventricular Dysfunction

	Training group (n = 18)		Control group (n =9)	
	Before	After	Before	After
Fiber size (μm)				
Type I	58 ± 8	72 ± 8*	64 ± 10	65 ± 7
Type II	71 ± 8	83 ± 9*	68 ± 8	69 ± 7
Fiber type (%)				
Type I	18 ± 7	20 ± 8	20 ± 8	22 ± 9
Type II	82 ± 7	80 ± 8	80 ± 9	78 ± 7
Volume density of mitochondria (vol %)	4.8 ± 0.8	5.9 ± 0.8*	4.3 ± 1.2	4.5 ± 0.9

* p < .001 vs. before training.

Reprinted from *Journal of the American College of Cardiology*, 26, Belardinelli R, Georgiou D, Scocco V, Barstow TJ, Purcaro A, Low intensity exercise training in patients with chronic heart failure, 979, Copyright 1995, with permission from the American College of Cardiology.

study changes in skeletal muscle inorganic phosphate and phosphocreatine ratios resulting from exercise training in chronic heart failure patients. Minotti and colleagues (1990) used a wrist flexor exercise program with incremental wrist exercise testing performed pre- and post-training. Importantly, exercise training did not increase heart rate or cardiac output and constituted pure local muscle training. The trained forearm increased in endurance by approximately 260% (no change in endurance for the untrained forearm). With incremental exercise testing, the inorganic phosphate/phosphocreatine ratio was reduced, consistent with less phosphocreatine depletion and an increase in oxidative capacity of the forearm.

Stratton et al. (1994) used isometric handgrip exercise training and incremental weight pulley exercise testing in 10 patients with chronic heart failure. After training, exercise testing duration increased 19% and the rate of resynthesis of phosphocreatine and ATP improved. Less depletion of phosphocreatine and a higher pH during exercise were also observed.

Adamopoulos and associates (1993) studied the responses to calf muscle plantar flexion exercise testing and training in chronic heart failure patients and control subjects. Before exercise training, phosphocreatine depletion, the decrease in pH, and the increase in ADP during exercise testing were all greater in patients than in the normal controls. After training, calf plantar flexion exercise capacity improved. Although no change in pH during exercise testing after training was found, phosphocreatine depletion had improved (although still greater than controls), and its recovery time was significantly shorter (0.56 versus 0.89 min). These three studies demonstrate that local muscle oxidative capacity is impaired in chronic heart failure and may be improved by exercise training. The impairment may be due, in part, to deconditioning.

Magnusson and coworkers (1996) sought to train one muscle group with strengthening exercise. A single-leg knee extension exercise, four sets of 6-10 repetitions at 80% of maximal dynamic strength, was performed three times per week for eight weeks in five CHF patients. Quadriceps muscle cross-sectional area increased 9% and maximal strength by 40%. Therefore, local muscle training may be helpful in these patients in terms of both aerobic capacity and muscular strength and deserves further investigation.

Diastolic function is impaired in patients with left ventricular dysfunction. Belardinelli et al. (1995a) assessed diastolic filling variables with Doppler echocardiography in 55 patients with idiopathic dilated cardiomyopathy with a mean LVEF of approximately 20%. Thirty-six patients were randomized to exercise training with the remaining 19 serving as nonexercise controls. Exercise training took place three times per week on cycle ergometers at an intensity of 60% of $\dot{V}O_2$peak. After two months of exercise, patients in the training group demonstrated improvements in the following diastolic function variables: rapid filling fraction, peak filling rate, early peak filling velocity, and the E/A ratio (where E = peak velocity of early diastolic filling wave, and A = peak velocity of late filling). An unexpected finding was that only patients with an abnormal relaxation pattern on their echocardiographic assessment of diastolic function demonstrated a significant improvement in $\dot{V}O_2$peak with training. This finding requires confirmation by other data before firm conclusions may be drawn regarding its importance. The number of subjects with abnormal relaxation was small (n = 12) and other studies have demonstrated the importance of peripheral adaptations to exercise training in heart failure patients in achieving a training effect. However, these data do suggest that it may be possible to predict which patients may improve aerobic capacity with short-term exercise training. A second randomized, controlled trial from Belardinelli and colleagues (1996a) confirmed the improvement in peak early filling rate and peak filling rate after training. The $\dot{V}O_2$peak improved by a mean of 15% due to an increase in a-$\bar{v}O_2$ difference. Cardiac index was unchanged with training.

Wilson and associates (1996) demonstrated with hemodynamic monitoring that some CHF patients exhibit a normal cardiac output response to exercise and that others do not. They reported that patients with a normal cardiac output response to exercise were more likely to improve $\dot{V}O_2$peak by at least 10% (11 of 21 patients in their study) than were patients with an abnormal cardiac output response (1 of 11 of these patients).

Hertzeanu and colleagues (1993) investigated the effects of exercise training on ventricular arrhythmias and neurohormonal activation in chronic heart failure patients with coronary artery disease and large myocardial infarctions (many with anterior location). The study was not randomized, but three groups of patients were included: Group I = patients who performed arm ergometry; Group II = patients who performed calisthenic exercises; and Group III = control patients who received no rehabilitation exercise. Holter monitoring (24-hour) and measurement of plasma neurohormones were performed at baseline and after 24 months. Isolated premature ventricular contractions and nonsustained ventricular tachycardia were more prevalent in nonrehabilitated patients. In addition, plasma norepinephrine and atrial naturetic peptide were lower in the rehabilitated patients (-146 pg/ml for norepinephrine; -230 pg/ml for atrial naturetic peptide) (Shemesh et al. 1995). Thus, relatively long-term exercise rehabilitation (two years) of patients with ischemic left ventricular dysfunction may reduce the arrhythmogenic effect of neurohormones as well as the incidence of ventricular arrhythmias.

This group of investigators pioneered the use of arm ergometer training for chronic heart failure patients. Typically, their patients perform arm exercises for 30 minutes at an intensity of 70% of maximal workload on a twice weekly basis. They have reported average increases in arm exercise capacity of approximately 30% (Kellerman 1990).

Jugdutt and colleagues (1988) urged caution in recommending exercise training for patients with moderate-sized anterior wall Q-wave myocardial infarctions who exhibit left ventricular asynergy (akinesia or dyskinesia) of 18% or more. After a very mild 3-month exercise program that began 15 weeks after MI, these patients demonstrated more cardiac shape distortion, expansion, and wall thinning. The LVEF and functional capacity also worsened. Other investigators who have studied patients with large MIs have not observed adverse effects on LVEF or ventricular volumes related to exercise training status (Rowe et al. 1989; Goebbels et al. 1997). In a randomized controlled trial, Giannuzzi and associates (1992) evaluated the effects of six months of cycle ergometry on left ventricular function and shape in 49 men who had a first Q-wave anterior wall MI. Patients had LVEFs > 25% and started the study approximately six weeks after their MI. Exercise tests and echocardiograms were performed at the beginning of the study and after six months of training. Cycling exercise was performed three times weekly at an intensity of 80% of peak heart rate for 30 minutes per session. Subjects in the exercise and control groups with LVEFs of < 40% exhibited some degree of left ventricular enlargement, regional dilation, and shape distortion. These investigators expanded the trial to include 75 patients (Giannuzzi et al. 1994). For patients with LVEFs < 40%, end-diastolic volume increased significantly in the original and the exercise and control groups; left ventricular enlargement was less pronounced in the trained subjects. End-systolic volume increased in controls, but not in the exercise group. Although patients with reduced left ventricular function after Q-wave anterior wall MI tend to experience adverse left ventricular remodeling over time, exercise training appears to be beneficial in limiting progressive deterioration in left ventricular function.

Dubach and associates (1997b) used magnetic resonance imaging to assess left ventricular remodeling with exercise in a randomized, controlled trial containing subjects with ischemic cardiomyopathy. No adverse effects on left ventricular size or function were found after two months of exercise training.

These data notwithstanding, some authorities continue to question the potential adverse effects on left ventricular size of long-term exercise training as a result of elevated wall stress during activity (McKelvie et al. 1995). Demopoulos and associates (1997) evaluated the fitness benefits and left ventricular wall stress of lower intensity training in 16 patients with chronic heart failure (either ischemic or nonischemic etiology, mean LVEF 21%). Patients cycled (semirecumbent posture) for 60 minutes, four sessions

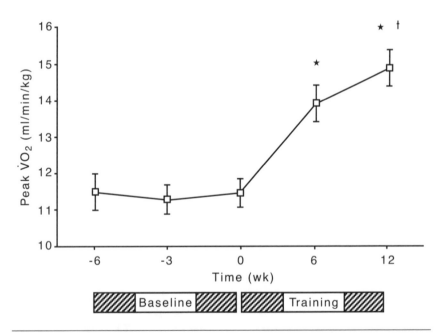

Figure 4.15 $\dot{V}O_2$peak measured 6 and 3 weeks and immediately before low-level exercise training and after 6 and 12 weeks of training. ★ $p < .001$ vs. baseline, † $p < .005$ vs. 6 weeks.

per week at an intensity of   50% $\dot{V}O_2$peak (measured on the semirecumbent cycle) for 12 weeks. Right heart catheter measurements of pulmonary
capillary wedge pressure and echocardiographic determination of left ventricular diastolic wall stress were performed in nine patients during cycle
exercise corresponding to   50% (intensity of training used in their study)
and 70% to 80% of $\dot{V}O_2$ peak (more conventional training intensity for CHF
patients). As figure 4.15 illustrates, $\dot{V}O_2$ peak measured on three occasions
prior to training was stable. With training, $\dot{V}O_2$ peak increased from 11.5
± 0.4 (baseline) to 14.0 ± 0.5 and 15.0 ± 0.5 ml/kg/min, respectively, at six
and 12 weeks (p < .001 versus baseline). Figure 4.16 demonstrates a significantly lower pulmonary capillary wedge pressure and left ventricular diastolic wall stress during exercise at   50% $\dot{V}O_2$ peak intensity than with exercise at conventional intensity. Again, this study demonstrates clearly that
low intensity exercise results in fitness gains for patients with severe CHF.

In an extremely novel approach, Meyer and colleagues (1996a, 1996b,
1997a, 1997b) studied the effects of high-intensity interval exercise training

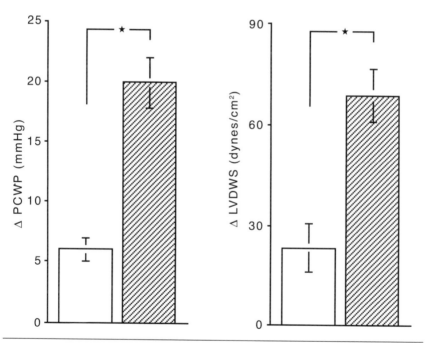

Figure 4.16   Changes in pulmonary capillary wedge pressure (PCWP) and left
ventricular diastolic wall stress (LVDWS) during exercise at   50% (open bars)
and 70% to 80% of $\dot{V}O_2$peak (hatched bars). ★ p < .01.

in patients with severe CHF. They devised a steep ramp cycle exercise test (three minutes unloaded pedaling followed by intensity increments of 25 watts each 10 seconds) to assess leg power, and studied various combinations of exercise intensity and work/rest intervals. Patients also performed a standard ramp cycle exercise test. Figure 4.17 shows the steep ramp test and the exercise intensity and work/rest interval combination that the investigators found to be most suitable: 30 second work-60 second recovery (pedaling at 15 watts) intervals at an intensity of 50% of the maximal watts attained during the steep ramp test. The steep ramp and the standard ramp exercise tests elicited similar cardiovascular responses in terms of peak heart rate and blood pressure. The $\dot{V}O_2$peak and blood lactate were slightly greater for the standard ramp test. However, the peak cycle power was 250% greater for the steep ramp test (200 watts vs. 79 watts). Training was performed five times per week for a cycling duration of 15 minutes. Each week the steep ramp test was repeated and the work interval intensity increased accordingly. In addition to cycling, treadmill walking (three times

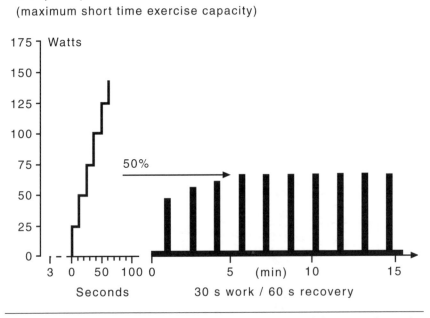

Figure 4.17 Schematic of the steep ramp exercise test and the interval exercise regimen. The first three work intervals served as a warm-up for the 50% of maximum watts intensity chosen for the program.

Reprinted, with permission, from MeyerK, Samek L, Schwaibold M, Westbrook S, Hajric R, Beneke R, Lehmann M, Roskamm H. 1997. Interval training in patients with severe chronic heart failure: Analysis and recommendations for exercise procedures. *Med Sci Sports Exerc* 29(3):306-312.

per week, 10 minutes per session) with intervals of 60 seconds fast pace (mean speed 2.4 mph) and 60 seconds active recovery (mean speed 0.9 mph) were performed. After three weeks of training, mean $\dot{V}O_2$peak increased from 12.2-14.6 ml/kg/min (p < .001). These investigators reasoned that the interval training approach would stimulate skeletal muscle adaptation with the high intensity work interval while minimizing cardiac stress. Figure 4.18 compares exercise intensity and selected exercise variables during interval training and at a reference exercise intensity of 75% of $\dot{V}O_2$peak derived from a standard ramp cycle exercise test. As can be seen, the cardiopulmonary and neurohormonal responses to the interval training were very similar to those for 75% of $\dot{V}O_2$peak, although the work interval intensity was 240% higher. Thus, brief interval exercise at relatively high intensities appears to be an alternative approach to exercise training in CHF patients. However, further work needs to be performed assessing the acute and

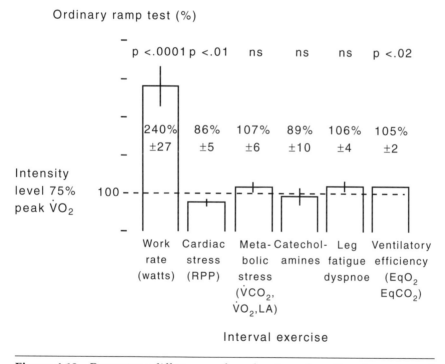

Figure 4.18 Percentage differences of work rate and cardiopulmonary and neurohormonal variables during interval training and standard exercise training at 75% of $\dot{V}O_2$peak (100 = intensity at 75% $\dot{V}O_2$peak).

Reprinted, with permission, from Meyer K, Samek L, Schwaibold M, Westbrook S, Hajric R, Beneke R, Lehmann M, Roskamm H. 1997. Interval training in patients with severe chronic heart failure: Analysis and recommendations for exercise procedures. *Med Sci Sports Exerc* 29(3):306-312.

chronic effects of high-intensity interval exercise on left ventricular size and function.

One investigation of exercise training after large myocardial infarction complicated by ventricular aneurysm is available in the literature. Giordano et al. (1988) exercise trained 60 patients with a definite left ventricular aneurysm (echocardiographic determination) four days per week for a total of fifty minutes at an intensity of 70% to 80% of maximal heart rate. Fifty-two of the patients had experienced an anterior wall infarction and the mean LVEF was 39% (25 patients had LVEFs of < 35%). No training-related problems occurred and average peak cycle workload during graded exercise testing improved after training. Pulmonary artery hemodynamic monitoring during rest and exercise demonstrated no change in left ventricular filling pressure at rest or during exercise.

Muscle metabolic abnormalities are found in respiratory as well as skeletal muscles of patients with chronic heart failure. Mancini et al. (1995) investigated the effects of selective respiratory muscle training on symptoms and exercise capacity of 14 patients (eight with idiopathic dilated cardiomyopathy, six with ischemic LV dysfunction; mean LVEF 22%). All of the patients were current nonsmokers and all took ACE inhibitors. Three months of training, three times per week for approximately 90 minutes, included the following:

- Isocapneic hyperpnea
- Resistive breathing with an inspiratory muscle trainer
- Maximal inspiratory and expiratory effort
- Abdominal muscle strengthening exercises

Before and after the 12-week period of training, graded exercise testing with analysis of expired air, pulmonary function testing, a six-minute walk, and the maximal sustainable ventilatory capacity (the maximal level of isocapneic hyperpnea that can be sustained for 12 minutes) was accomplished. Six patients dropped out of the study for nonmedical reasons and constituted a nonrandomized control group. No improvements in any of the variables were observed for the control subjects. Patients who trained their respiratory musculature exhibited the following improvements:

- Increased maximal inspiratory pressure (+24 cm H_2O)
- Increased maximal expiratory pressure (+58 cm H_2O)
- Increased maximal sustainable ventilatory capacity (+28 L/min)
- Increased six-minute walk distance (+319 m)
- Increased $\dot{V}O_2$ peak (+2 ml/kg/min)
- Improved symptoms of dyspnea

This study, although somewhat limited by a small number of participants and nonrandomized design, suggests that respiratory muscle training may be very beneficial for selected heart failure patients. Furthermore, by focusing on a relatively small muscle mass during training, respiratory training may be well tolerated by patients with very limited cardiovascular exercise capacities. Additional studies of the clinical utility of such training are needed.

Kavanagh and associates (1996) demonstrated important improvements in quality-of-life variables, such as a reduction in dyspnea and fatigue, improved emotional status, and better adjustment to disability in only four weeks of exercise training. These benefits persisted over 52 weeks of program participation.

Since exercise training does improve aerobic capacity and reduces neurohormonal activation, there are theoretical reasons to expect the clinical benefits of reduced cardiac events and mortality. Three investigations involving patients with ischemic left ventricular dysfunction have addressed the effects of training on morbidity and mortality. Belardinelli and coworkers (1996b) randomized 42 patients to exercise or control groups and followed both groups for approximately 18 months. The exercise group improved VO_2 peak by a mean of 26% and had less myocardial ischemia assessed with thallium perfusion scanning. At follow-up, 17 patients had experienced cardiac events, but the trained group had a significantly lower percentage of patients with events (19% vs. 75%, $p < .01$). Specchia and associates (1996) randomized a large (n = 256), heterogeneous group of postmyocardial infarction patients to exercise training or control groups. For patients with LVEFs of < 41%, the relative risk of cardiac death in a control group patient was 8.63 times that of the trained group. Risk of death was similar for both groups in patients with LVEFs > 40%. Belardinelli's group (1997) expanded their 1996 study to 88 subjects using a similar experimental design. Again, major cardiac events (over two years) occurred more frequently in the control group (47%) than in exercise training patients (18%). The change in VO_2peak with training was an independent predictor of a better outcome. For patients with ischemic left ventricular dysfunction, exercise training appears to reduce cardiac events and cardiac death.

Summary of Potential Benefits of Exercise Training for Patients With Chronic Heart Failure

The data presented in this section of the chapter provide strong evidence in favor of exercise training for patients with left ventricular dysfunction. Several benefits of habitual physical activity may be expected (although not all patients will receive all benefits). Patients may experience beneficial increases or improvements in the following:

- VO_2peak

- Physical work capacity and submaximal exercise endurance
- Leg blood flow
- Arterial oxygen content
- Maximal cardiac output
- Spontaneous daily activity
- Skeletal muscle aerobic enzyme activity
- Skeletal muscle fiber size
- Skeletal muscle endurance
- Skeletal muscle strength (with resistance training)
- Phosphocreatine and ATP resynthesis
- Ventilatory anaerobic threshold
- Parasympathetic nervous system activity
- Diastolic function
- Respiratory muscle function (with specific respiratory muscle training)
- Morbidity and mortality (patients with coronary artery disease)
- Quality-of-life indices

Also, patients may develop beneficial decreases in the following factors:

- Symptoms of dyspnea, fatigue, weakness
- Submaximal exercise $\dot{V}_E$ and $\dot{V}CO_2$
- Submaximal exercise respiratory exchange ratio
- Neurohormonal activation
- Sympathetic nervous system activity
- Rest heart rate
- Submaximal exercise blood lactate concentration
- New York Heart Association functional class
- Ventricular arrhythmias
- Phosphocreatine depletion during isometric exercise
- Submaximal exercise heart rate

Studies show that no change occurs in the following variables:

- Pulmonary artery pressure
- Mean arterial pressure during exercise
- Pulmonary capillary wedge pressure
- Right atrial pressure
- Left ventricular end-diastolic pressure

- Left ventricular end-systolic volume
- Left ventricular end-diastolic volume
- Left ventricular ejection fraction
- Submaximal exercise $\dot{V}O_2$

Home exercise training as well as supervised training has been shown to be both safe and effective in short-term training studies. Regional factors such as the availability of supervised programs, and patient characteristics (for example, patient or family confidence, history of symptomatic ventricular arrhythmias, exercise capacity, etc.) may largely determine whether patients are allowed to exercise alone or with medical supervision.

This chapter has demonstrated many important and beneficial adaptations to exercise training for patients with myocardial ischemia or left ventricular dysfunction. Even in these high-risk cardiac patients, training is safe if proper selection and exclusion criteria are followed. The next chapter provides practical suggestions for the development of exercise training programs for these patients.

References

Adamopoulos S, Coats AJS, Brunotte F, Arnolda L, Meyer T, Thompson CH, Dunn JR, Stratton J, Kemp GJ, Radda GK, Rajagopalan B. 1993. Physical training improves skeletal muscle metabolism in patients with chronic heart failure. *J Am Coll Cardiol* 21:1101-1106.

Adamopoulos S, Piepoli M, Meyer T, Barlow C, Radaelli A, Kremastinos D, Sleight P, Poole-Wilson P, Coats A. 1995. Physical training in patients with chronic heart failure: Overview and predictors of training-induced improvement in exercise tolerance. *Circulation* 92(Suppl I):541.

Ades PA, Grunvald MH, Weiss RM, Hanson JS. 1989. Usefulness of myocardial ischemia as predictor of training effect in cardiac rehabilitation after acute myocardial infarction or coronary bypass grafting. *Am J Cardiol* 63:1032-1036.

Ades PA, Waldmann ML, Poehlman ET, Gray P, Horton ED, Horton ES, LeWinter MM. 1993. Exercise conditioning in older coronary patients: Submaximal lactate response and endurance capacity. *Circulation* 88:572-577.

Arvan S. 1988. Exercise performance of the high-risk acute myocardial infarction patient after cardiac rehabilitation. *Am J Cardiol* 62:197-201.

Belardinelli R, Georgiou D, Cianci G, Berman N, Ginzton L, Purcaro A. 1995a. Exercise training improves left ventricular diastolic filling in patients with dilated cardiomyopathy: Clinical and prognostic implications. *Circulation* 91:2775-2784.

Belardinelli R, Georgiou D, Cianci G, Purcaro A. 1996a. Effects of exercise training on left ventricular filling at rest and during exercise in patients with ischemic cardiomyopathy and severe left ventricular systolic dysfunction. *Am Heart J* 132:61-70.

Belardinelli R, Georgiou D, Cianci G, Purcaro A. 1996b. Prognostic significance of exercise training of moderate intensity in patients with coronary artery disease and left ventricular systolic dysfunction. *Circulation* 94:I-327.

Belardinelli R, Georgiou D, Cianci G, Purcaro A. 1997. Prognostic significance of moderate exercise training in chronic heart failure. *J Am Coll Cardiol* 29:425A.

Belardinelli R, Georgiou D, Scocco V, Barstow TJ, Purcaro A. 1995b. Low intensity exercise training in patients with chronic heart failure. *J Am Coll Cardiol* 26:975-982.

Blumenthal JA, Rejeski WJ, Walsh-Riddle M, Emery CF, Miller H, Roark S, Ribisl PM, Morris PB, Brubaker P, Williams RS. 1988. Comparison of high- and low-intensity exercise training after acute myocardial infarction. *Am J Cardiol* 61:26-30.

Clausen JP, Trap-Jensen J. 1970. Effects of training on the distribution of cardiac output in patients with coronary artery disease. *Circulation* 42:611-624.

Coats AJS. 1993. Exercise rehabilitation in chronic heart failure. *J Am Coll Cardiol* 22(Suppl A):172-177.

Coats AJS, Adamopoulos S, Meyer TE, Conway J, Sleight P. 1990. Effects of physical training in chronic heart failure. *Lancet* 235:63-66.

Coats AJS, Adamopoulos S, Radaelli A, McCance A, Meyer TE, Bernardi L, Solda PL, Davey P, Ormerod O, Forfar C, Conway J, Sleight P. 1992. Controlled trial of physical training in chronic heart failure: Exercise performance, hemodynamics, ventilation, and autonomic function. *Circulation* 85:2119-2131.

Conn EH, Williams RS, Wallace AG. 1982. Exercise responses before and after physical conditioning in patients with severely depressed left ventricular function. *Am J Cardiol* 49:296-300.

Demopoulos L, Bijou R, Fergus I, Jones M, Strom J, LeJemtel TH. 1997. Exercise training in patients with severe congestive heart failure: Enhancing peak aerobic capacity while minimizing the increase in ventricular wall stress. *J Am Coll Cardiol* 29:597-603.

Dubach P, Myers J, Dziekan G, Goebbels U, Reinhart W, Muller P, Buser P, Stulz P, Vogt P, Ratti R. 1997a. Effect of high intensity exercise training on central hemodynamic responses to exercise in men with reduced left ventricular function. *J Am Coll Cardiol* 29:1591-1598.

Dubach P, Myers J, Dziekan G, Goebbels U, Reinhart W, Vogt P, Ratti R, Muller P, Miettunen R, Buser P. 1997b. Effect of exercise training on myocardial remodeling in patients with reduced left ventricular function after myocardial infarction: Application of magnetic resonance imaging. *Circulation* 95:2060-2067.

Ehsani AA, Biello DR, Schultz J, Sobel BE, Holloszy JO. 1986. Improvement of left ventricular contractile function by exercise training in patients with coronary artery disease. *Circulation* 74:350-358.

Ehsani AA, Martin WH, Heath GW, Coyle EF. 1982. Cardiac effects of prolonged and intense exercise training in patients with coronary artery disease. *Am J Cardiol* 50:246-254.

Ferguson RJ, Taylor AW, Cote P, Charlebois J, Dinelle Y, Perronet F, De Champlain J, Bourassa MG. 1982. Skeletal muscle and cardiac changes with training in patients with angina pectoris. *Am J Physiol* 243 (*Heart Circ Physiol* 12):830-836.

Foster C, Pollock ML, Anholm JD, Squires RW, Ward A, Dymond DS, Rod JL, Saichek RP, Schmidt DH. 1984. Work capacity and left ventricular function during rehabilitation after myocardial revascularization surgery. *Circulation* 69:748-755.

Franklin BA. 1991. Exercise training and coronary collateral circulation. *Med Sci Sports Exerc* 23:648-653.

Giannuzzi P, Temporelli PL, Corra U, Gattone M, Galli M, Marcassa C. 1994. Attenuation of unfavorable remodeling by long-term physical training in post-infarct patients with exertional ischemia and left ventricular dysfunction. *Circulation* 90(Suppl I):14.

Giannuzzi P, Temporelli PL, Tavassi L, Corra A, Gattone M, Imparato A, Giordano A, Schweiger C, Sala L, Maliverni C. 1992. Exercise in anterior myocardial infarction (EAMI): An ongoing multicenter randomized study. Preliminary results on left ventricular function and remodeling. *Chest* 101(Suppl):315-321.

Giordano A, Giannuzzi P, Tavazzi L. 1988. Feasibility of physical training in post-infarct patients with left ventricular aneurysm: A haemodynamic study. *Eur Heart J* 9:11-15.

Gobel AJ, Hare DL, Macdonald PS, Oliver RG, Reid MA, Worcester MC. 1991. Effects of early programmes of high and low intensity exercise on physical performance after transmural acute myocardial infarction. *Br Heart J* 65:126-131.

Goebbels U, Dziekan G, Myers J, Dubach P, Reinhart WH, Ratti R, Bremerich J, Bauser P, Muller P. 1997. Effect of exercise training in post-MI heart failure: One year follow-up with magnetic resonance imaging. *J Am Coll Cardiol* 29:378A.

Hagberg JM. 1991. Physiologic adaptations to prolonged high-intensity exercise training in patients with coronary artery disease. *Med Sci Sports Exerc* 23:661-667.

Hagberg JM, Ehsani AA, Holloszy JO. 1983. Effect of 12 months of intense exercise training on stroke volume in patients with coronary artery disease. *Circulation* 67:1194-1199.

Hambrecht R, Fiehn E, Niebauer J, Offner B, Riede U, Schuler G. 1995a. Two-year-follow-up of exercise training in patients with chronic heart failure: Effects on cardiorespiratory fitness and left ventricular function. *Circulation* 92(Suppl I):398.

Hambrecht R, Fiehn E, Yu J, Niebauer J, Weigl C, Hilbrich L, Adams V, Riede U, Schuler G. 1997. Effects of endurance training on mitochondrial ultrastructure and fiber type distribution in skeletal muscle of patients with stable chronic heart failure. *J Am Coll Cardiol* 29:1067-1073.

Hambrecht R, Niebauer J, Fiehn E, Kalberer B, Offner B, Hauer K, Riede U, Schlierf G, Kubler W, Schuler G. 1995b. Physical training in patients with stable chronic heart failure: Effects on cardiorespiratory fitness and ultra-structural abnormalities of leg muscle. *J Am Coll Cardiol* 25:1239-1249.

Hambrecht R, Niebauer J, Marburger C, Grunze M, Kalberer B, Hauer K, Schlierf G, Kubler W, Schuler G. 1993. Various intensities of leisure time physical activity in patients with coronary artery disease: Effects on cardio-respiratory fitness and progression of coronary atherosclerotic lesions. *J Am Coll Cardiol* 22:468-477.

Hartung GH, Rangel R. 1981. Exercise training in post-myocardial infarction patients: Comparison of results with high-risk coronary and post-bypass patients. *Arch Phys Med Rehab* 62:147-150.

Hertzeanu HL, Shemesh J, Aron LA, Aron AL, Peleg E, Rosenthal T, Metro M, Kellerman JJ. 1993. Ventricular arrhythmias in rehabilitation and nonrehabilitated post-myocardial infarction patients with left ventricular dysfunction. *Am J Cardiol* 71:24-27.

Jette M, Heller R, Landry F, Blumchen G. 1991. Randomized 4-week exercise program in patients with impaired left ventricular function. *Circulation* 84:1561-1567.

Jugdutt BI, Michorowski BL, Kappagoda CT. 1988. Exercise training after anterior Q wave myocardial infarction: Importance of regional left ventricular function and topography. *J Am Coll Cardiol* 12:362-372.

Kavanagh T, Myers MG, Baigrie RS, Mertens DJ, Sawyer P, Shephard RJ. 1996. Quality of life and cardiorespiratory function in chronic heart failure: Effects of 12 months' aerobic training. *Heart* 76:42-49.

Kellerman JJ, Shemesh J, Fisman EZ, Steinmetz A, Ben-Ari E, Drory Y, Lapidot C. 1990. Arm exercise training in the rehabilitation of patients with impaired ventricular function and heart failure. *Cardiology* 77:130-138.

Kennedy CC, Spiekerman RE, Lindsay MI Jr, Mankin HT, Frye RL, McCallister BD. 1976. One-year graduated exercise program for men with angina pectoris: Evaluation by physiologic studies and coronary angiography. *Mayo Clin Proc* 51:231-236.

Keteyian SJ, Levine AB, Brawner CA, Kataoka T, Rogers FJ, Schairer JR, Stein PD, Levine TB, Goldstein S. 1996. Exercise training in patients with heart failure: A randomized controlled trial. *Ann Intern Med* 124:1051-1057.

Kiilavuori K, Sovijarvi A, Naveri H, Ikonen T, Leinonen H. 1996. Effect of physical training on exercise capacity and gas exchange in patients with chronic heart failure. *Chest* 110:985-991.

Laslett LJ, Paumer L, Amsterdam EA. 1985. Increase in myocardial oxygen consumption indices by exercise training at the onset of ischemia in patients with coronary artery disease. *Circulation* 71:958-962.

Lee AP, Ice R, Blessy R, Sanmarco ME. 1979. Long-term effects of physical training on coronary patients with impaired ventricular function. *Circulation* 60:1519-1526.

Letac B, Cribier A, Desplanches JF. 1977. A study of left ventricular function in coronary patients before and after physical training. *Circulation* 56:375-378.

Magnusson G, Gordon A, Kaijser L, Sylven C, Isberg B, Karpakka J, Saltin B. 1996. High intensity knee extensor training in patients with chronic heart failure: Major skeletal muscle improvement. *Eur Heart J* 17:1048-1055.

Mancini DM, Hanson D, LaManca J, Donchez L, Levine S. 1995. Benefit of selective respiratory muscle training on exercise capacity in patients with chronic congestive heart failure. *Circulation* 91:320-329.

Martin WH 3rd, Ehsani AA. 1987. Reversal of exertional hypotension by prolonged exercise training in selected patients with ischemic heart disease. *Circulation* 76:548-555.

Martin WH 3rd, Heath G, Coyle EF, Bloomfield SA, Holloszy JO, Ehsani AA. 1984. Effect of prolonged intense endurance training on systolic time intervals in patients with coronary artery disease. *Am J Cardiol* 107:75-81.

McKelvie RS, Teo KK, McCartney N, Humen D, Montague T, Yusuf S. 1995. Effects of exercise training in patients with chronic heart failure: A critical review. *J Am Coll Cardiol* 25:789-796.

Meyer K, Samek L, Schwaibold M, Westbrook S, Hajric R, Beneke R, Lehmann M, Roskamm H. 1997a. Interval training in patients with severe chronic heart failure: Analysis and recommendations for exercise procedures. *Med Sci Sports Exerc* 29:306-312.

Meyer K, Samek L, Schwaibold M, Westbrook S, Hajric R, Lehmann M, Edfeld D, Roskamm H. 1996a. Physical responses to different modes of interval exercise in patients with chronic heart failure: Application to exercise training. *Eur Heart J* 17:1040-1047.

Meyer K, Schwaibold M, Westbrook S, Beneke R, Hajric R, Gornandt L, Lehmann M, Roskamm H. 1996b. Effects of short-term exercise training and activity restriction on functional capacity in patients with severe chronic congestive heart failure. *Am J Cardiol* 78:1017-1022.

Meyer K, Schwaibold M, Westbrook S, Beneke R, Hajric R, Lehmann M, Roskamm H. 1997b. Effects of exercise training and activity restriction on 6-minute walking test performance in patients with chronic heart failure. *Am Heart J* 133:447-453.

Minotti JR, Johnson EC, Hudson TL, Zuroske G, Murata G, Fukashima E, Cagle TG, Chick TW, Massie BM, Icenogle MV. 1990. Skeletal muscle response to exercise training in congestive heart failure. *J Clin Invest* 86:751-758.

Paterson DH, Shephard RJ, Cunningham D, Jones NL, Andrew G. 1979. Effects of physical training on cardiovascular function following myocardial infarction. *J Appl Physiol* 47:482-489.

Raffo JA, Luksic IY, Kappagoda CT, Mary DA, Whitaker W, Linden RJ. 1980. Effects of physical training on myocardial ischemia in patients with coronary artery disease. *Br Heart J* 43:262-269.

Redwood DR, Rosing DR, Epstein SE. 1972. Circulatory and symptomatic effects of physical training in patients with coronary artery disease and angina pectoris. *N Eng J Med* 286:959-965.

Rowe MH, Jelinek MV, Liddell N, Hugens M. 1989. Effect of rapid mobilization on ejection fractions and ventricular volumes after acute myocardial infarction. *Am J Cardiol* 63:1037-1041.

Schuler G, Schlierf G, Wirth A, Mautner HP, Scheurlen H, Thumm M, Roth H, Scharz F, Kohlmeier M, Mehmel HC, Kubler W. 1988. Low-fat diet and regular, supervised physical exercise in patients with symptomatic coronary artery disease: Reduction of stress-inducted myocardial ischemia. *Circulation* 77:172-181.

Shemesh J, Grossman E, Peleg E, Steinmetz A, Rosenthal T, Motro M. 1995. Norepinephrine and atrial naturetic peptide responses to exercise testing in rehabilitation and nonrehabilitated men with ischemic cardiomyopathy after healing of anterior wall myocardial acute myocardial infarction. *Am J Cardiol* 75:1072-1074.

Sinoway LI. 1988. Effect of conditioning and deconditioning stimuli on metabolically determined blood flow in humans and implications for congestive heart failure. *Am J Cardiol* 62:45E-48E.

Specchia G, DeServi S, Scire A, Assandri J, Berzuini C, Angoli L, LaRovere MT, Cobelli F. 1996. Interaction between exercise training and ejection fraction in predicting prognosis after a first myocardial infarction. *Circulation* 94:978-982.

Squires RW, Lavie CJ, Brandt TR, Gau GT, Bailey KR. 1987. Cardiac rehabilitation in patients with severe ischemic left ventricular dysfunction. *Mayo Clin Proc* 62:997-1002.

Stratton JR, Dunn JF, Adamopoulos S, Kemp GJ, Coats AJS, Rajagopalan B. 1994. Training partially reverses skeletal muscle metabolic abnormalities during exercise in heart failure. *J Appl Physiol* 76:1575-1582.

Sullivan MJ, Higginbotham MB, Cobb FR. 1988. Exercise training in patients with severe left ventricular dysfunction: Hemodynamic and metabolic effects. *Circulation* 78:506-515.

Sullivan MJ, Higginbotham MB, Cobb FR. 1989. Exercise training in patients with chronic heart failure delays ventilatory anaerobic threshold and improves submaximal exercise performance. *Circulation* 79:324-329.

Todd IC, Bradnam MS, Cooke MB, Ballantyne D. 1991. Effects of daily high-intensity exercise on myocardial perfusion in angina pectoris. *Am J Cardiol* 68:1593-1599.

Wilson JR, Groves J, Rayos G. 1996. Circulatory status and response to cardiac rehabilitation in patients with heart failure. *Circulation* 94:1567-1572.

CHAPTER 5

Exercise Programming Suggestions

This chapter provides information regarding exercise programming for patients with either substantial exercise-related myocardial ischemia or severe left ventricular dysfunction. Some patients will have both myocardial ischemia during exercise and severe left ventricular dysfunction and will not be candidates for either surgical revascularization or transplantation. These patients, as discussed previously, are at the highest risk for sudden cardiac death during exercise or at rest.

Exercise Intensity Prescription for Patients With Myocardial Ischemia

Exercise intensities above the ischemic threshold are not advised for patients with substantial amounts of exercise-induced ischemia. The risk of life-threatening ventricular arrhythmias and potential catecholamine-related thrombus formation is greater in the setting of ischemia. Target heart rates for patients with exercise-induced ischemia should be set at least 10 beats/min below the heart rate that corresponds to the ischemic threshold.

The ischemic threshold, from an exercise ECG standpoint, is defined as the heart rate (or rate-pressure product) that results in at least one mm of horizontal ST segment depression. The threshold may have corresponding anginal symptoms or may be painless (silent ischemia). The determination of the ischemic threshold in patients undergoing thallium, sestamibi, or exercise echocardiographic testing may be difficult if the exercise ECG does not show ST segment changes or is abnormal at rest, since these techniques provide identification and quantification of ischemia only at peak exercise. Radionuclide angiography with multigated acquisition of data allows determination of left ventricular ejection fraction with each exercise stage and thus allows for the determination of the ischemic threshold independent of the exercise ECG. Since most laboratories use semi-supine cycle exercise for radionuclide angiographic studies, the heart rate-systolic blood pressure relationship is altered from that of upright exercise. The heart rate tends to be lower and the systolic blood pressure higher with supine versus upright exercise. Use of the rate-pressure product at the ischemic threshold for exercise intensity prescription is a useful technique and will be the focus of one of the case examples discussed later in the chapter.

The ischemic threshold is not necessarily always present at a given heart rate or rate-pressure product (Hatcher et al. 1995). Changes occur in coronary perfusion from increased or decreased coronary vasoconstriction. Blood levels of anti-ischemic medications are not constant. Transient platelet aggregation may occur and reduce coronary flow. Therefore, ECG monitoring during at least the first several exercise sessions in patients with severe exertional myocardial ischemia is warranted. For patients with exercise-related ischemia, repeated exercise bouts separated by short rest periods appear to reduce the severity of ischemia observed in later exercise bouts (Stewart et al. 1995; Maybaum et al. 1996). This may represent warm-up or ischemic preconditioning (repeated brief episodes of ischemia that protect the myocardium from further ischemic damage). These data provide a rationale for interval approaches (exercise bouts of short duration interspersed with brief rest periods) for patients with substantial ischemia. In addition, since some evidence indicates that platelet aggregation occurs more frequently during exercise at intensities greater than the ventilatory anaerobic threshold than below, exercise intensity for patients with ischemia should be prescribed below the threshold (Chicharro et al. 1994).

Symptoms of angina or anginal equivalent may be helpful in prescribing exercise for high-risk patients. Avoidance of angina is recommended for patients with extensive areas of myocardial ischemia. Use of prophylactic nitroglycerine is prudent for patients who have painful ischemia during exercise training sessions. Careful education of patients regarding the proper taking of anti-ischemic medications is extremely important. One-a-day beta-blocking drugs do not demonstrate a consistent effect on exercise heart rate over a 24-hour period and patients should be advised that the heart rate response to exercise may vary depending upon the interval between the time of taking the medication and the time of the exercise session. Missing a dose of anti-ischemic medication prior to an exercise session is obviously not recommended.

Patients with painless ischemia must be able to accurately self-monitor heart rate, if they are not on ECG telemetry, during exercise training. For patients who are unable to self-monitor, ECG monitoring in a supervised program or the use of an accurate electronic pulse monitor is advised. The issue of medically supervised versus nonsupervised exercise training of high-risk patients is discussed later in this chapter.

Prescription of exercise mode, duration, frequency, and progression of training for patients with ischemia follow the same general guidelines as for patients with chronic heart failure. Excellent additional references for exercise prescription are available (American College of Sports Medicine 1995; Pollock et al. 1995; Pashkow and Dafoe 1993).

Exercise Programming for Patients With Chronic Heart Failure

The following topics of exercise prescription for heart failure patients are presented:

- Medical evaluation
- Graded exercise testing
- Prescription of exercise intensity
- Modes of exercise
- Exercise duration, frequency, and progression
- Exercise program pearls
- Safety issues: supervised versus nonsupervised training
- What is the optimal level of supervision of exercise programs for high-risk cardiac patients?
- Case examples

Medical Evaluation

Patients with depressed left ventricular function require a thorough evaluation by a physician (preferably a cardiologist) before beginning an exercise program. The specific evaluation may vary from physician to physician but usually includes a comprehensive cardiovascular examination, ECG, chest x-ray, blood analyses (electrolytes included), and a measure of left ventricular function (for example, echocardiogram or rest radionuclide angiogram). As with all patients who begin exercise programs, a musculoskeletal exam may be indicated for patients with osteoarthritis or other orthopedic problems. Heart failure must be well compensated. The following are contraindications to exercise testing and training: uncompensated heart failure, rales, uncontrolled edema, uncontrolled arrhythmias, symptoms at rest or with minimal exertion (class IV), unstable angina, resting sinus tachycardia (> 120 beats/min) or hypotension (systolic blood pressure < 90 mmHg), or hypokalemia (serum potassium < 3.0 mEq/L).

Neither patients with left ventricular ejection fractions of < 20% nor patients with large anterior wall myocardial infarctions should be excluded from exercise training if no contraindication is present.

Graded Exercise Testing

Exercise testing for the purpose of determining exercise capacity, heart rate and blood pressure response, cardiac rhythm, symptoms, and the presence of myocardial ischemia is invaluable in the exercise prescription process. As was discussed in chapter 4, analysis of expired air adds greatly to the precision of determination of aerobic capacity and is extremely helpful in exercise prescription. Again, the relationship between rest LVEF and $\dot{V}O_2$ peak is not easily predicted and patients with low LVEFs, without contraindications, may safely undergo symptom-limited exercise testing.

For patients with directly measured aerobic capacities of < 2 METs (< 7 ml O_2/kg/min), exercise training is difficult. Walking on the treadmill at 1 mph requires a $\dot{V}O_2$ of approximately 2 METs. These patients require one-on-one supervision by a knowledgeable exercise professional with an interval approach to training. Arm and leg calisthenic exercises while seated in a chair or very slow cycle ergometry may be tolerated by these patients. Such patients are often hospitalized and receive inotropic support while awaiting transplantation, if appropriate.

Occasionally, patients with poor left ventricular function who have not undergone graded exercise testing for a variety of reasons are referred for exercise training. In this situation, a supervised ECG and blood pressure-monitored program is essential at the outset of training to document the appropriateness of heart rate, blood pressure, and symptomatic responses to exercise. In effect, the monitored exercise sessions serve as a rudimentary form of exercise testing.

Prescription of Exercise Intensity

In general, exercise intensity for patients with left ventricular dysfunction should begin conservatively, given that most patients have below normal exercise capacities and are deconditioned (Hanson 1994). The American College of Sports Medicine guidelines (1995) for exercise prescription provide a framework for prescription of intensity based upon aerobic capacity.

For patients with exercise capacities below 3 METs, initial intensity of 40% to 50% of $\dot{V}O_2$ peak is adequate. Target heart rates using the heart rate reserve method may be given (see the case examples discussed later in the chapter). For patients with atrial fibrillation, target heart rates are not generally useful. The heart rate corresponding to the desired percentage of VO_2 peak may also be used, as well as perceived exertion ratings of 11-13 on the original Borg scale. Patients should avoid angina and excessive fatigue or dyspnea. If exercise capacity is >3 METs, the initial training intensity may be set at 50% to 60% of capacity. This corresponds to approximately 12-14 on the Borg scale (see table 5.1). After several weeks of training, most patients with chronic heart failure may increase exercise intensity to 60% to 70% of VO_2peak.

Table 5.1   Borg Rating of Perceived Exertion Scale

6	
7	Very, very light
8	
9	Very light
10	
11	Fairly light
12	
13	Somewhat hard
14	
15	Hard
16	
17	Very hard
18	
19	Very, very hard
20	

Reprinted, by permission, from *Borg's Perceived Exertion and Pain Scales* by G. Borg, 1998, Champaign, IL: Human Kinetics.

Modes of Exercise

For patients with very limited exercise tolerance, nonweight-bearing activities such as cycle ergometry should be considered initially. An activity such as cycling with no or minimal external resistance allows for a very low exercise-energy expenditure. This type of activity is particularly advisable for patients with obesity. Additional popular forms of exercise for chronic heart failure patients include walking (treadmill, track, shopping mall or school, out-of-doors), recumbent cycling, stair climbing, combination arm-leg cycle ergometer, cross-country ski simulator, water exercise or swimming, and arm ergometry. Some patients with left ventricular dysfunction have the ability to walk/jog or jog continuously.

Since many patients with chronic heart failure have prolonged oxygen uptake kinetics at the onset and offset of exercise, as has been previously described, careful attention to gradual warm-up and cool-down is very important. Five to ten minutes of warm-up and cool-down low-intensity activity is recommended, although the duration of this activity may be shortened for patients with very poor exercise capacities.

Exercise Duration, Frequency, and Progression

Patients with exercise capacities of < 3 METs are capable of only short bouts of exercise and an interval approach to their training is recommended. Interval training allows a greater training volume to be performed with less fatigue, especially for very deconditioned patients. Table 5.2 provides an example of an interval exercise approach that may be used with these

Table 5.2   Initial Interval Exercise Prescription and Progression in Patients With Chronic Heart Failure

A. Exercise capacity (EC) < 3 METs

Week	%EC	Total min	Min ex	Min rest	Reps
1	50	10-15	3-5	3-5	3-4
2	50	12-20	5-7	3-5	3
3	50-60	15-25	7-10	3-5	3
4	50-60	20-30	10-15	2-3	2
5	60-70	25-40	12-20	2	2
6	60-70	30-45	15-25	2	1-2

B. Exercise capacity 3-5 METs

Week	%EC	Total min	Min ex	Min rest	Reps
1	50-60	15-20	7-10	2-3	3
2	50-60	20-30	10-15	2	2
3	60-70	25-40	15-20	2	2
4	60-70	30-45	20-30	2	1-2

Min = minutes; Ex = exercise; Reps = repetitions.

Reprinted, by permission, from American College of Sports Medicine. *ACSM's Guidelines for Exercise Testing and Prescription.* 5th ed. Baltimore:Williams & Wilkins. 1995.

patients. Ideally, two or three daily sessions of exercise are performed with a gradual progression of exercise duration and intensity.

For patients with aerobic capacities of 3-5 METs, frequency should be set at one or two sessions daily with an initial duration of three to 10 minutes (see table 5.2). Patients with exercise capacities of > 5 METs may begin with 10 minutes of exercise with a frequency of at least three sessions per week, although in my experience, a frequency of 5-6 sessions per week is much more beneficial in improving exercise capacity. For all patients with chronic heart failure, the duration of exercise should be gradually increased (5-15 minutes per week) with a goal of 30 minutes to as much as 60 minutes with a frequency of four to six sessions per week. Not all patients, however, particularly the elderly and those with poor exercise capacities, will progress to this volume of training.

Repeat graded exercise testing after 2-3 months is helpful in assessing the amount of improvement in exercise capacity and in updating the exercise prescription. It should be noted that some patients may dramatically improve submaximal exercise endurance and yet demonstrate only a small or no increase in $\dot{V}O_2$ peak.

Many patients with chronic heart failure are extremely sedentary and deconditioned. In addition, heart failure appears to result in skeletal muscle metabolic abnormalities independent of disuse, as discussed previously. The result for some patients is skeletal muscle atrophy and associated weakness that may make routine tasks of lifting and carrying difficult for them. A modest program of isotonic strengthening exercise using handheld weights (1-5 pounds), commercial weight training machines, or elastic resistance bands may be very beneficial. Our group previously documented only modest heart rate and systolic blood pressure responses during mild weight training with commercial machines in cardiac patients, some with depressed left ventricular function (Squires et al. 1991b). Selecting a resistance so that the patient can perform 15-20 repetitions of each exercise without straining is well tolerated by many heart failure patients. Several investigations of the safety and benefit of weight training for patients with chronic heart failure are currently underway.

As reviewed in chapter 4, a novel high-intensity, short duration interval training program has been designed, investigated, and reported by Meyer and Roskamm (1997). This approach will likely become another accepted method for exercise programming for CHF patients.

Exercise Program Pearls

Since environmental extremes increase demands on cardiac function, patients with chronic heart failure should be cautioned to avoid exercise in hot/humid or cold weather conditions. Patients must dress appropriately for the prevailing weather conditions if outdoor activity is performed. Moderate altitude may pose a particular problem for patients with ischemic left ventricular dysfunction and requires modification of activity (Squires 1985).

In order to avoid further reduction in already impaired skeletal muscle blood flow, patients should wait at least one hour after a meal before performing exercise.

Medications scheduled for morning usage should be taken before morning exercise. However, some patients may experience a greater likelihood of hypotension during exercise if they take vasodilators immediately prior to their exercise session.

Patients should choose an exercise time of day when they feel at their best. Most patients with chronic heart failure seem to better tolerate morning exercise rather than afternoon sessions.

Patients should weigh themselves daily. A > 4-pound weight gain over 1-2 days may indicate early cardiac decompensation. However, some patients experience a temporary increase in fluid volume (probably plasma) at 2-6 weeks after beginning an exercise training program (Sullivan 1994). This can be managed by increasing the diuretic dosage and following the patient carefully for other adverse signs or symptoms. Hypotension at rest and an increase in resting heart rate of > 10 beats/min may also indicate decompensation.

For patients taking diuretics, occasional checks of blood potassium concentration are an important consideration to guard against hypokalemia.

Patients must be watched for the following exercise-related signs of worsening heart failure:

- Excessive dyspnea with exercise
- Exertional hypotension
- Lightheadedness
- Sustained arrhythmias
- New onset exertional angina
- Excessive fatigue during or after exercise

Patients have good and bad days with day-to-day variability in exercise performance in terms of endurance and symptoms.

Safety Issues: Supervised Versus Nonsupervised Training

The previous chapters have provided a scientific basis for the recommendation of prudent exercise training for appropriately selected patients who, because of severe left ventricular dysfunction or large amounts of exercise-induced myocardial ischemia, are considered at high risk for cardiac death and serious exercise-related complications. None of the investigations of exercise training for these types of patients discussed previously has demonstrated an unacceptable complication rate associated with exercise. A few of the studies followed patients for 35-42 months (Squires et al 1987;

Lee et al. 1979), but the majority of investigations lasted only a few months. There are no randomized, controlled trials specifically investigating the effect of long-term exercise training on rates of rehospitalization, utilization of health care resources, or cardiac mortality. However, it is my feeling, as well as the opinion of others who have worked extensively with high-risk cardiac patients, that the benefits of exercise training far outweigh the risks.

Several prominent medical organizations have published guidelines for the recommended level of medical supervision during exercise training for high-risk patients, including the following:

The American College of Cardiology (1986) recommends ECG monitoring during exercise training for these patients:

- LVEFs < 30%
- Resting complex ventricular arrhythmias (Lown type 4 or 5)
- Ventricular arrhythmias appearing or increasing with exercise
- Decrease in systolic blood pressure with exercise
- Survivors of sudden cardiac death
- Postmyocardial infarction patients with complications of congestive heart failure, cardiogenic shock, or serious ventricular arrhythmias
- Patients with marked exercise-induced ischemia
- Inability to self-monitor heart rate

The American College of Physicians (1988) position paper on rehabilitation services essentially is equivalent to these recommendations.

While these guidelines are specific, they are now over ten years old. In addition, insurance coverage for long-term ECG-monitored exercise training is not available for most patients.

The American Association of Cardiovascular and Pulmonary Rehabilitation (1995) recommends that high-risk patients receive close monitoring, but does not define what is meant by monitoring.

The American College of Sports Medicine (1995) recommends that high-risk patients should attend clinically supervised programs.

The American Heart Association (Fletcher et al. 1995) recommends that high-risk patients should be supervised with ECG and blood pressure monitoring during exercise training until the safety of training is established, 6-12 sessions or more, as necessary.

Ideally, high-risk cardiac patients should begin exercise training with some degree of medical supervision. The optimal type and intensity of supervision are not known. Supervision of exercise training includes the following potential factors:

- Exercise prescription, including proper warm-up and cool-down procedures, knowledge of the target heart rate (and ability to self-monitor heart rate) and perceived exertion range, knowledge of symptoms of exertional intolerance and the recommended patient response to symptoms, prudent progression of the amount of exercise, knowledge of the effect of environmental factors on exercise training, etc.

- Familiarization with appropriate exercise equipment
- Direct instruction and supervision of exercise sessions by qualified personnel, as in a cardiac rehabilitation program
- Monitoring of the ECG and blood pressure during exercise training
- Periodic adjustment of the exercise prescription based on changes in the clinical situation
- Medical intervention during serious exercise-related complications such as prolonged angina, life-threatening ventricular arrhythmias, heart failure decompensation

All of this supervision may be accomplished in a modern cardiac rehabilitation program. However, estimates of participation rates of patients with coronary artery disease in cardiac rehabilitation programs in the United States range from 11% to 38% of eligible patients (Agency for Health Care Policy and Research 1995). Participation of patients with chronic heart failure unrelated to coronary artery disease is estimated to be much less, given the fact that Medicare and most major third party payers currently do not fund supervised exercise programs for these patients. Many patients cannot afford to pay out-of-pocket for long-term supervised exercise programs. There is a need to develop low-cost, medically supervised exercise programs in many areas of North America.

Several potential models of differing levels of supervision of exercise training for high-risk cardiac patients are conceivable. These include models A-E, which are described below:

- Model A: Direct supervision of exercise sessions (three or more per week) by qualified staff in a medical institution (no unsupervised training allowed in this model); ECG monitoring on an individual patient-need basis
- Model B: Partial direct supervision of long-term exercise training by medical personnel with one to three supervised sessions/week plus additional unsupervised sessions (at home or community exercise facility)
- Model C: Initial medical supervision for a period of days to weeks with a subsequent unsupervised long-term program
- Model D: Initial medical supervision for a period of days to weeks with subsequent unsupervised long-term exercise training with periodic supervised exercise sessions (every one to three months)
- Model E: Initial medical supervision with subsequent home exercise

program monitored by telephone contact with an established cardiac rehabilitation program (voice contact and ECG-monitoring capability)

Squires and associates (1991a) reported the use of transtelephonic supervision of exercise training sessions for 67 patients, four of whom had ischemic or idiopathic dilated cardiomyopathy. The patients averaged 27 exercise sessions. Although no serious medical emergencies occurred during the study, the availability of accessing the emergency medical system in the patients' locality by the medical professional providing the supervision supplied an additional measure of safety for these patients.

Patients who exercise at home should only do so if someone is in the immediate area in order to respond in the event of a medical emergency. In the event of cardiac collapse, CPR is effective only if promptly followed by rapid defibrillation. Activation of the emergency medical system by a family member and the response time of the emergency team are of critical importance. Recently, external semiautomatic cardioverter-defibrillators have been shown to be effective when used in the field by nonmedical persons such as the police (White 1996). In the event of a cardiac collapse, these devices require only that adhesive electrodes be placed on the victim's chest. The device then determines if an arrhythmia is present and prompts the user to activate the device for automatic defibrillation or cardioversion, as is necessary. In the future these relatively low-cost (approximately $2,000) devices conceivably could be placed (with appropriate training) with the significant others of high-risk patients who exercise at home. The same considerations for activation of the emergency medical system in response to cardiac collapse are necessary for patients who choose to exercise at a nonmedically supervised community exercise facility.

Monitoring of the ECG during exercise training sessions for high-risk patients is routine in most centers, at least for the first few weeks of the program. However, few studies have addressed the benefits of such monitoring. Keteyian and associates (1995) reviewed their experience with ECG monitoring in 289 consecutive patients, 80 considered at high risk by American College of Cardiology criteria, during an average of 14 exercise sessions. The high-risk patients did have more minor events (angina, nonsustained arrhythmias) during training sessions than did the lower risk patients. However, the frequency of new onset, asymptomatic events that were discovered only by ECG monitoring, was 3.8% for both high-risk and lower risk patients. Whether a longer program of ECG-monitored exercise training would provide more compelling data for the clinical benefit of monitoring is not known at present. The issue of the benefit of continuous ECG monitoring during exercise sessions for high-risk patients requires more study before definitive guidelines may be given. Individualization of the use of monitoring is obviously important, and local patterns of practice will also influence the use of monitoring.

Patients with a history of primary (not in the setting of an acute myocardial infarction) malignant ventricular arrhythmias such as sudden cardiac death due to ventricular tachycardia or fibrillation, or symptomatic ventricular tachycardia, are a special population of high-risk patients that deserve further discussion. Many of these patients have severe left ventricular dysfunction. For survivors of sudden cardiac death, one- and three-year mortality is approximately 25% and 40%, respectively (Osborn 1996). Use of an implantable cardioverter-defibrillator (ICD) for selected patients with sudden cardiac death who have no effective drug treatment, or for patients with hemodynamically unstable ventricular tachycardia that is not controlled with drugs, reduces one- and three-year mortality to approximately 1.6% and 3%, respectively. Patients with ICDs who experience shocks have a higher mortality, 5% to 20% at one year, although most deaths are due to worsening heart failure or electromechanical dissociation, and are not sudden.

Data regarding exercise training in patients with life-threatening ventricular arrhythmias are sparse. Exercise may exert an arrhythmogenic effect due to increased sympathetic nervous system tone, release of catecholamines from the adrenal medulla, and potential myocardial ischemia as discussed by Kelly (1995). This investigator studied 42 patients who were recently hospitalized for evaluation and treatment of malignant ventricular arrhythmias. These patients participated in 1,246 ECG-monitored exercise sessions as part of their treatment. Thirty percent of the patients exhibited nonsustained ventricular tachycardia, but there were no deaths or life-threatening emergencies. Four episodes of increasing ventricular tachycardia and three episodes of symptomatic ventricular tachycardia were discovered during the exercise sessions.

What Is the Optimal Level of Supervision of Exercise Programs for High-Risk Cardiac Patients?

There are no clear guidelines available to answer this question, at present. Practice patterns may differ by geographic location. The availability and scope of supervised exercise programs is not uniform across North America. However, the following considerations for the intensity of supervision are provided, based on the literature, as well as the author's clinical experience.

In my experience, patients with a history of primary sudden cardiac death or hemodynamically unstable ventricular tachycardia, and who do not receive an ICD, are best served by a medically supervised cardiac rehabilitation exercise program with continuous ECG monitoring for at least some of the exercise sessions (model A). This recommendation is based on the extremely high mortality for this population. Patients with ICDs may exercise without direct medical supervision and ECG monitoring after they have demonstrated the ability to perform their exercise prescription in an appropriate manner.

Other high-risk patients should be entered into cardiac rehabilitation programs following the American Heart Association model of direct medical supervision, including continuous ECG and periodic blood pressure monitoring, until the stability of the patient as well as the safety of the exercise prescription for the individual patient has been determined, usually after at least 6-12 sessions (model D). Alternative use of transtelephonic supervision (voice and periodic ECG monitoring) of home exercise training is an option (model E).

For patients who have participated in a series of supervised exercise sessions and who have graduated to unsupervised training, periodic recheck appointments with health care professionals, specifically addressing the exercise program, are strongly encouraged. Monitored exercise sessions at the rehabilitation facility on a quarterly basis seem to be effective in this regard.

At my institution, we see a number of high-risk cardiac patients who live outside of the immediate geographic area. Our approach for these patients includes performance of a cardiopulmonary exercise test, a consultation with the patient and significant others to provide the exercise prescription, and ideally, one or more supervised, monitored exercise sessions for the patient to become familiar with the exercise program, and referral to a supervised exercise program in the patient's home location. If a supervised program is not available, a home or unsupervised community exercise center program is recommended, with availability of telephone contact with health professionals from our program.

Case Examples: Exercise Prescription and Risk Factor Management for High-Risk Cardiac Patients

The following issues require careful consideration before initiating exercise training for high-risk cardiac patients:

- Clinical status of the patient
- Graded exercise testing responses
- Exercise prescription specifics
- Safety concerns: the need for medical supervision with or without continuous ECG monitoring during exercise training, warning signs and symptoms, availability of emergency medical services

Case Study Number One

Myocardial Ischemia With Electrocardiographic ST Segment Depression and Typical Angina Pectoris

This patient is a 69-year-old married man (height 173 cm, weight 64 kg) who is a retired, licensed practical nurse. Currently he works six hours, four or five days a week, bagging groceries at a food market.

Past Medical History

Steroid-dependent asthma for several decades.

Cardiovascular History

Developed chest tightness December 1 and promptly reported to the emergency room of his local hospital. An acute inferior wall myocardial infarction was diagnosed and treated with thrombolysis (streptokinase), aspirin, metoprolol (subsequently stopped due to exacerbation of asthma symptoms), and isosorbide dinitrate.

A thallium treadmill exercise test was performed December 4 to 11.3 minutes on the Naughton protocol (estimated 5 METs), with an increase in heart rate from 72-140 beats/min and in blood pressure from 90/50 to 110/50. The test was terminated due to 3 out of 4 angina and 2+ mm of horizontal ST segment depression (leads V4 to V6). The thallium perfusion images demonstrated a moderate-sized inferior-inferoseptal scar and a moderate-sized area of severe anterior-anteroseptal ischemia.

On December 5, a coronary angiogram revealed a left ventricular ejection fraction of 57% with severe hypokinesis of the posterobasal and posterolateral segments. Coronary artery anatomy included significant obstructive lesions in the mid left anterior descending (80%), first diagonal branch (85%), mid circumflex (two lesions: 70% and 60%), and the distal right coronary artery (70%). The vessels were not amenable for coronary angioplasty and bypass surgery was recommended but refused by the patient.

Medical Management

The patient was prescribed the following medications:

Prednisone 15 mg qd

Albuterol 2.5 mg q4h

Isosorbide mononitrate 60 mg qd

Aspirin 81 mg qd

Cardiac Rehabilitation Consultation

The patient was seen December 6, prior to hospital dismissal. Coronary risk factors were identified and included the following:

Age

Gender

Marked family history (father, two brothers, sister, 55-70 years at time of MI or CABG)

Recent blood lipids included a low-density lipoprotein cholesterol (LDL-C) concentration of 85 mg/dl and a high-density lipoprotein cholesterol (HDL-C) of 71 mg/dl.

Diet was fairly prudent, the patient had never been a smoker, and was moderately physically active (yard work, regular leisurely walking). The patient and spouse did not attribute the development of coronary artery disease to stress or other psychosocial factors. The patient was moderately knowledgeable regarding coronary disease due to his former profession and experience with other family members with the disease.

The patient will be encouraged to attend all of the patient education classes dealing with coronary artery disease, see the dietitian with his wife for a specific plan in this regard, and attend the patient and spouse support group. Psychological assessment will be done with the Symptom Checklist 90-R instrument (a pencil and paper assessment of psychological status that patients may complete by themselves, with subsequent scoring and interpretation by a psychologist). The blood lipids are at goal presently and will be repeated in approximately three months. At that time, a plasma homocysteine level will be obtained and treatment with folic acid and vitamins B6 and B12 will be recommended if the concentration is > 10 μmol/L.

Risk Stratification for Exercise Training

Three-vessel coronary disease with good left ventricular systolic function; considerable exercise-induced myocardial ischemia. Overall risk: moderate to high

Cardiac Rehabilitation Models

Model B (ideal), D, or E

Exercise Prescription

The intensity of exercise will be prescribed using a target heart rate range of 108-120 beats/min (50% to 70% of heart rate reserve), perceived exertion ratings of 12-14 (somewhat hard), keeping the intensity below anginal symptoms and with less than 1 mm of ST segment depression. Pre-exercise sublingual nitroglycerine will be recommended if angina occurs predictably with exercise training. A supervised, ECG-monitored program with three sessions per week for approximately two weeks will be followed by an unmonitored phase III exercise program with home exercise sessions (goal frequency 4-6 sessions/week). Initial exercise duration will be ten minutes progressing to 30-45 minutes per session (increase of 3-5 minutes per session, as tolerated). Exercise modes will be walking, cycle ergometry (including arm and leg ergometry), and upper extremity strengthening exercise with handheld weights.

Return to work will occur in approximately four weeks, if the patient can exercise at an intensity of 4-5 METs without angina and ST segment depression.

Case Study Number Two

Symptomatic and Electrocardiographically Silent Substantial Myocardial Ischemia

This patient is a 56-year-old married man who owns and operates a scrap yard business.

Past Medical History

Noncontributory.

Cardiovascular History

In 1989, the patient developed chest pain that resulted in coronary artery bypass surgery (left internal mammary artery to left anterior descending (LAD) artery; saphenous vein to right coronary artery (RCA)). Recurrent chest pain resulted in a coronary angiogram in 1994 that revealed a patent graft to the LAD, an occluded graft to the RCA, and a subtotal occlusion of the mid circumflex artery that was treated successfully with balloon angioplasty.

Chest pressure led to an emergency room evaluation on November 10 of this year with a diagnosis of a non-Q-wave myocardial infarction. An echocardiogram in the emergency room demonstrated a left ventricular ejection fraction of 53% and severe hypokinesis of the inferior wall.

An emergency angiogram was performed and revealed a patent graft to the LAD, graft occlusion to the RCA, and the following significant lesions: a 90% proximal LAD, 100% proximal RCA, collaterals from the LAD to the RCA, 90% mid RCA, and a 95% mid circumflex. Balloon angioplasty was successfully performed on the circumflex lesion.

A thallium treadmill exercise study was performed five days later to 7.3

minutes of the Bruce protocol (estimated 8 METs), with an increase in heart rate from 69-99 beats/min and in blood pressure from 126/80 to 132/88, with an endpoint of general fatigue. There were no electrocardiographic changes with exercise, and the patient denied anginal symptoms. However, the perfusion images showed a large area of severe apical, septal, and inferior wall ischemia with a fixed inferolateral defect consistent with infarction.

The patient opted for medical treatment rather than further attempts at revascularization. Medications (taken at the time of the thallium treadmill test) included the following:

Atenolol 100 mg qAM

Isosorbide dinitrate 30 mg tid

Nifedipine XL 60 mg qAM

Aspirin 81 mg qd

Lovastatin 40 mg qhs

Cholestyramine 2 packets bid

Cardiac Rehabilitation Consultation

The patient was seen approximately two weeks after hospital dismissal. Coronary risk factors were discussed and included the following:

Gender

Significant mixed hyperlipidemia (recent total cholesterol 306 mg/dl, LDL-C 192 mg/dl, HDL-C 41 mg/dl, triglycerides 365 mg/dl, on medications and a prudent diet)

Family history (father with MI at 51 years)

Past cigarette use (22 pack-years, stopped in 1989)

Sedentary lifestyle

Obesity (waist/hip = 1.10, weight 106 kg, height 178 cm)

The patient and spouse will be asked to see the dietitian for weight loss and blood lipid nutritional advice. Consideration of altering the patient's lipid medication with the possible change to atorvastatin 20 mg qd will be undertaken. A repeat blood lipid profile will be done in six to eight weeks. Although the patient does not have a history of hypothyroidism, a sensitive thyroid stimulating hormone level, and a fasting blood glucose will also be measured at that time to rule out potential secondary causes for the patient's dyslipidemia. A goal weight of approximately 90 kg will be suggested.

A psychological assessment will be carried out with the Symptom Checklist 90-R, with possible referral to a psychologist or psychiatrist, if indicated. Patient and spouse will be encouraged to attend the support group and classes dealing with coronary artery disease.

Risk Stratification for Exercise Training
Silent, substantial ischemia, three-vessel coronary atherosclerosis with well-preserved left ventricular function. Overall risk: moderate to high

Cardiac Rehabilitation Models
Model B (ideal), D, or E

Exercise Prescription
The initial program should be supervised with ECG monitoring for a period of two to four weeks, four to five sessions/week (to facilitate weight loss) until the responses of the patient have been adequately observed and the patient is capable of self-monitoring. The immediate problem in prescribing exercise intensity for this patient is the lack of data regarding the ischemic threshold: no ST segment changes, no anginal symptoms, evidence for severe exercise-induced ischemia at peak exercise but no perfusion information for submaximal exercise intensities (thallium perfusion data are only available for peak exercise, not for submaximal exercise stages). The patient's heart rate reserve from the thallium treadmill test was 30 beats/min. Arbitrarily, an initial target heart rate of 10 beats/min above the resting heart rate corresponding to perceived exertion ratings of 11-13 (fairly light to somewhat hard) was prescribed. Pre-exercise sublingual nitroglycerine use was suggested. Exercise duration will begin at 10 minutes (not including warm-up and cool-down activities) and gradually increase (2-5 minutes per session, as tolerated) to a goal of 45-60 minutes (weight loss emphasis). Treadmill walking and cycle ergometry will be the modes of exercise training for this patient. If feasible, an exercise radionuclide angiogram will be performed in several weeks to assess ischemia during each submaximal exercise stage (see case study number 11 for an example of the data derived from this test).

Case Study Number Three

Ischemic Cardiomyopathy With No Evidence of Reversible Ischemia
The patient is a 71-year-old married, retired man.

Past Medical History
Seizure disorder, 1976, currently treated and quiescent; peripheral vascular disease of the lower extremities (post two surgical revascularization procedures in 1993 and 1995), presently mild right calf claudication; hyperten-

sion; chronic obstructive lung disease, chronic bronchitis, requires oxygen during waking hours.

Cardiovascular Disease History

Anteroseptal myocardial infarction in 1989 with resultant severe left ventricular dysfunction, multiple hospitalizations for congestive heart failure.

Recent evaluation by a cardiologist with the following test results:

Echocardiogram: moderate left ventricular enlargement, severe decrease in systolic function, left ventricular ejection fraction 15%; best preserved function in the basal septum and the basal segments of the remaining walls; all other walls are akinetic; mild left atrial enlargement with mild mitral regurgitation

Dipyridamole thallium scan: increased pulmonary uptake; large area of infarction involving the entire apex, anterior wall, septum, inferior wall, and lateral wall, probable apical aneurysm; no evidence of reversible ischemia

Pulmonary function: mild airflow limitation with FEV_1 2.32 L (80% of normal); severely reduced diffusing capacity (8.1 ml/min/mmHg, 33% of normal) with a P_aO_2 of 76.5 mmHg

Coronary angiography: 70% left main; 100% mid left anterior descending; 80% mid circumflex; 50% mid right coronary artery; patent saphenous vein bypass to the distal right coronary artery, patent left internal mammary implant to the first obtuse marginal

Cardiopulmonary exercise test (performed without supplemental oxygen): 5.4 minutes to an exercise intensity of 2.0 mph, 14% grade; heart rate increased from 69-116 beats/min, blood pressure from 118/80 to 132/72; ECG was nondiagnostic for ischemia secondary to a left bundle branch block on the resting ECG; no significant arrhythmias; limiting symptom of dyspnea; VO_2 peak of 938 ml/min, 14.3 ml/kg/min, 4.0 METs (59.6% of normal for age); plateau in the VO_2 curve noted, consistent with severe cardiac limitation to exercise; elevated ventilatory equivalent for CO_2 and decrease in arterial oxygen saturation (95% at rest, 88% at peak exercise) consistent with chronic pulmonary disease

Blood analyses: hemoglobin 12.5 gm/dl; potassium 3.8 mEq/L; total cholesterol 159 mg/dl, high-density lipoprotein cholesterol 39 mg/dl, low-density lipoprotein cholesterol 112 mg/dl, triglycerides 50 mg/dl

The patient was not felt to be a candidate for further revascularization. Medications consisted of the following:

Captopril 25 mg tid

Carbamazepine 200 mg tid

Phenytoin 100 mg tid

Digoxin 0.125 mg qd

Aspirin 81 mg qd

Furosemide 80 mg bid

Potassium 40 mEq qd

Coumadin 5 mg qd

Oxygen 2 L/min per nasal cannula

Cardiac Rehabilitation Consultation

The patient was seen approximately one week after hospital dismissal for assessment of coronary risk factors and for the feasibility of a structured exercise program. Coronary risk factors included the following:

Age

Gender

Cigarette smoking (42 pack-years, stopped in 1989)

Family history (father and brother with coronary deaths in their 60s)

The patient followed a very low-fat diet fanatically and walked at a slow pace 10-15 minutes daily with symptoms of mild dyspnea and mild right calf claudication. Blood lipids were close to the National Cholesterol Education Program for patients with documented atherosclerosis. A psychological profile will be obtained using the Symptom Checklist 90-R with possible referral to a mental health professional, pending the results. Education regarding coronary artery disease as well as chronic heart failure will be accomplished via classes and consultations with the patient and spouse. Attendance at the support group will be encouraged.

Risk Stratification for Exercise Training

Severely depressed left ventricular systolic function with multiple episodes of congestive failure, poor exercise capacity. Overall risk: high

Cardiac Rehabilitation Models

Model B (ideal) or D

Exercise Prescription

ECG-monitored phase II-type program with 3-4 supervised sessions/week for approximately four weeks, until the patient's exercise responses are determined to be appropriate and the patient's self-monitoring skills are adequate. The patient should then enter a nonmonitored, but medically supervised phase III-type program on a permanent basis with some home exercise sessions, as well. Cycle ergometry and treadmill walking will form the basis of the exercise program. Later, mild strengthening exercises for the upper and lower extremities (weight machines and handheld weights) will be added, as tolerated. A target heart rate range of 96-102 beats/min, which corresponds to 50% to 60% of measured $\dot{V}O_2$ peak, will be prescribed initially. Perceived exertion ratings of 11-13 (fairly light to somewhat hard) will also be used to establish an acceptable training intensity. Exercise duration will commence at 15 minutes per session, increasing by 1-3 minutes per session to a goal of 30-45 minutes. Intervals of exercise at 5-10 minutes duration will be used if the patient is unable to reach a continuous exercise duration of less than 30 minutes after two weeks in the program. Arterial oxygen saturation will be continuously monitored during the first few exercise sessions to ensure a saturation of > 88% with the use of supplemental oxygen. In approximately three months, a repeat exercise test (cardiopulmonary or radionuclide angiogram) will be considered to reassess the patient's responses to the exercise training program.

Case Study Number Four

Idiopathic Dilated Cardiomyopathy With an Extremely Poor Exercise Capacity

This patient is a 39-year-old married male computer analyst (height 178 cm, weight 115.7 kg).

Past Medical History

Type A hemophilia (mild), obesity, glucose intolerance (recent fasting blood glucose 113 mg/dl).

Cardiovascular History

Bicuspid aortic valve with significant stenosis resulting in aortic valve replacement surgery (tissue prosthesis) in 1988. Left ventricular ejection fraction 45% at that time.

The patient developed shortness of breath and was evaluated within the past month by a cardiologist with the following findings and treatment:

Echocardiogram: normal aortic tissue prosthesis, dilated left ventricle, global severe hypokinesis with a left ventricular ejection fraction of 15%

Cardiac catheterization: normal coronary arteries, increased left ventricular end-diastolic pressure consistent with moderate pulmonary hypertension. The patient was started on lisinopril 10 mg qd and digoxin 0.25 mg qd.

Cardiopulmonary exercise test: 2.9 minutes of treadmill exercise to 2.0 mph, 7% grade with limiting symptoms of dyspnea and general fatigue; heart rate increased from 99-160 beats/min, blood pressure increased from 114/70 to 130/64; the electrocardiogram was nondiagnostic for ischemia secondary to left bundle branch block, no significant arrhythmias were observed; $\dot{V}O_2$peak was 1.3 L/min, 11.0 ml/kg/min, 3.1 METs (27.2% of age and gender predicted maximum); respiratory exchange ratio 1.39; normal arterial oxygen saturation, 95% at rest, 92% at peak exercise; normal ventilatory variables

Cardiac Rehabilitation Consultation

The patient was referred for potential exercise training and follow-up, pending the decision of listing for cardiac transplantation. The exercise test results were compatible with a near-maximal effort by the patient and profound exertional intolerance. A portion of the exercise intolerance may be attributable to obesity and deconditioning. However, the findings are consistent with a severe cardiac output limitation to exercise.

The patient and spouse will be encouraged to see the dietitian for instruction in a low-fat, low-sodium, reduced calorie diet for weight loss from a current 116 kg to approximately 100 kg. Chronic heart failure education will be provided by the heart failure RN. Support group attendance will also be encouraged. Psychological assessment will be performed with the Symptom Checklist 90-R.

Risk Stratification for Exercise Training

Markedly below normal LVEF, extremely poor $\dot{V}O_2$ peak. Overall risk: very high

Cardiac Rehabilitation Models

Model A or B ideally; D or E (depending upon the circumstances)

Exercise Prescription

The patient will enter an ECG-monitored phase II exercise program with three to four supervised exercise sessions per week for approximately four to six weeks, until he can exercise continuously for 30 minutes at an energy expenditure of 4 METs. When that goal is achieved, the patient will continue in a supervised, but not monitored, phase III exercise program with at least two home exercise sessions per week with a total weekly exercise session frequency of 5 or 6. A target heart rate range of 132-144 beats/min (corresponding to 50% to 65% of measured $\dot{V}O_2$ peak) will be used, along with perceived exertion ratings of 11-13 (fairly light to somewhat hard) to regulate intensity of effort. The modes of activity will be cycle ergometry (standard and combination arm and leg), treadmill walking and low-level upper extremity strengthening with handheld weights. Initially, exercise intervals of 3-5 minutes with rest intervals of 2-3 minutes will be used with a total duration of 10-15 minutes at the outset (not including warm-up and cool-down activities). The total length of the training sessions will increase to 30-45 minutes, with a gradual increase in the length of the exercise intervals until the patient is able to exercise continuously for the entire 30-

45 minute session. A repeat cardiopulmonary exercise test will be performed in two to three months to reassess fitness and to refine the exercise prescription.

Case Study Number Five

Idiopathic Nondilated Cardiomyopathy

The patient is a 37-year-old married female secondary school teacher (height 158 cm, weight 52 kg).

Past Medical History

Irritable bowel syndrome.

Cardiovascular History

A "heart murmur" was detected by the patient's primary physician during an examination prompted by the symptom of increasing dyspnea with exertion. Referral to a cardiologist revealed a diagnosis of probable heart failure based upon the physical findings. An echocardiogram demonstrated normal left ventricular dimensions, mild mitral valve regurgitation and profound, global hypokinesis with a left ventricular ejection fraction of 10%. Pulmonary artery systolic pressure was elevated at 61 mmHg (pulmonary hypertension), and the left side filling pressures were elevated consistent with diastolic dysfunction.

Cardiac catheterization was performed with no evidence of coronary artery obstructive disease. A right ventricular biopsy did not find any evidence of an infiltrative myocardial disease. The diagnosis of idiopathic nondilated cardiomyopathy was made and digoxin 0.25 mg qd and captopril 12.5 mg tid was begun.

Cardiac Rehabilitation Consultation

The patient was referred for cardiopulmonary exercise testing and an exercise program. Treadmill exercise time was 5.3 minutes to an intensity of 2.0 mph and 14% grade with a limiting factor of fatigue. Heart rate increased from 85-137 beats/min and blood pressure from 108/80 to 116/84. The electrocardiogram revealed right bundle branch block with repolarization abnormalities consistent with digoxin therapy. With exercise, no meaningful ECG changes or arrhythmias were seen. The $\dot{V}O_2$peak was 842 ml/min, 16.2 ml/kg/min, or 4.6 METs, which was only 39% of age and gender expected consistent with a severe cardiac output limitation to exercise. Respiratory exchange ratio at peak exercise was 1.24, consistent with a near-maximal effort by the patient. There was no evidence of pulmonary limitation and arterial oxygen saturation was normal (97% at rest, 95% at peak exercise).

The patient was felt to be a candidate for potential transplantation, but was also encouraged to begin a progressive exercise training program. Patient and spouse education will involve chronic heart failure topics. Support group participation will be encouraged. Psychological evaluation will be performed as discussed in the previous cases.

Risk Stratification for Exercise Training
Profoundly low left ventricular ejection fraction; poor $\dot{V}O_2$peak. Overall risk: high

Cardiac Rehabilitation Models
Model B (ideal), D, or E

Exercise Prescription
An ECG-monitored program (phase II) will be recommended for four to six weeks, then an unmonitored, but supervised exercise program (phase III) will follow indefinitely with at least two unsupervised home exercise sessions per week (total frequency five to six sessions per week). Modes of activity will be cycle ergometry (including upper extremities), treadmill and free walking, upper extremity strengthening exercises with handheld weights. Exercise duration will commence at 10 minutes (excluding warm-up and cool-down) and gradually increase to 30-45 minutes per session. Alternatively, an interval program of 3-4 repeats of 8-10 minutes could be used, if fatigue makes continuous exercise of longer than 10 minutes difficult. A target heart rate range of 108-120 beats/min (corresponding to 50% to 60% of measured $\dot{V}O_2$ peak) and perceived exertion ratings of 11-14 (fairly light to somewhat hard) will be used. In three months, a repeat cardiopulmonary exercise test will be performed to evaluate progress and update the exercise prescription.

Case Study Number Six

Hypertrophic Cardiomyopathy With Pulmonary Hypertension

This patient is a 47-year-old married woman who works as an executive for a large marketing firm (height 162 cm, weight 51 kg).

Past Medical History
Noncontributory.

Cardiovascular History

The patient has carried a diagnosis of hypertrophic cardiomyopathy (HOCM) for the past eight years, resulting from an evaluation for symptoms of palpitations, dyspnea on exertion, and fatigue. One episode of paroxysmal atrial fibrillation has been documented.

She is able to work full-time and can walk slowly for several blocks, but presented for a cardiology evaluation because of increasing fatigue and dyspnea. Medications include the following:

Propranolol 80 mg bid

Verapamil LA 240 mg qd

Furosemide 20 mg qhs

Estrogen 0.625 mg qd

Progesterone 2.5 mg qd

An echocardiogram revealed classic hypertrophic cardiomyopathy with a basal septal thickness of 16 mm and a 100 mmHg outflow gradient from the left ventricular apex to the ascending aorta. Cardiac catheterization demonstrated normal coronary arteries, mild mitral regurgitation, and pulmonary hypertension with a pulmonary artery systolic pressure of 75-85 mmHg.

Cardiac Rehabilitation Consultation

The patient was referred for a cardiopulmonary exercise test and consideration for an exercise program, pending the decision regarding potential treatment options of permanent pacing versus myectomy (surgical removal of part of the basal septum to decrease the outflow gradient).

Treadmill exercise time was 3.8 minutes to a speed of 2.0 mph and a grade of 7.0%. Heart rate increased from 59-108 beats/min and the blood pressure response was flat at 90-100 mmHg systolic, and 50-60 mmHg diastolic. The electrocardiogram revealed no significant arrhythmias. Slight cyanosis of the fingernails was observed, although arterial oxygen saturation measured by oximetry decreased only from 96% at rest to 92% at peak exercise (mild desaturation). The ventilatory equivalent for carbon dioxide ($\dot{V}_E/\dot{V}CO_2$) was elevated at peak work (57), consistent with pulmonary hypertension. The $\dot{V}O_2$peak was only 564 ml/min, 11.3 ml/kg/min or 3.2 METs (35.9% of age and gender predicted). Respiratory exchange ratio was consistent with a good patient effort (R = 1.21). These results were consistent with a severe cardiac output limitation to exercise.

Risk Stratification for Exercise Training

Extremely poor exercise capacity; hypertrophic cardiomyopathy with a severe left ventricular outflow obstruction. Overall risk: high

Cardiac Rehabilitation Models

Model A (for the first several weeks), B (ideal for the long-term)

Exercise Prescription

For the first four to six weeks, the patient will exercise with close monitoring due to the increased risk of arrhythmic death and hypotensive blood pressure response during exercise secondary to HOCM. At that time, if the patient's responses are appropriate and the exercise intensity is > 3 METs during the exercise training sessions, the patient will be moved to a nonmonitored phase III program with at least two supervised exercise sessions per week supplemented with home exercise for a total frequency of 5 exercise sessions per week. Exercise mode will begin with treadmill walking and cycle ergometry (including the upper extremities). Intensity of exercise will be set using perceived exertion levels of 11-14 (fairly light to somewhat hard), a target heart rate range of 84-90 beats/min (corresponding to 50% to 60% of $\dot{V}O_2$ peak), and an adequate systolic blood pressure increase over rest during exercise (keep systolic blood pressure above pre-exercise levels). Since only mild arterial desaturation during exercise was noted during the exercise test, saturation during exercise training sessions will not be monitored. A repeat cardiopulmonary exercise test will be performed in 2-3 months to determine the patient's improvement in fitness and to refine the exercise prescription.

Case Study Number Seven

Severe Aortic Stenosis

This patient is a 79-year-old married, retired man (height 175 cm, weight 89.8 kg).

Past Medical History

Hypertension, chronic obstructive lung disease as a result of cigarette smoking (56 pack-years, stopped in 1987)

Cardiovascular History

Aortic stenosis (mild by echocardiographic assessment) was documented in 1990. The patient recently sought a consultation with a cardiologist for progressive dyspnea on exertion accompanied by mild angina. The evaluation resulted in the following findings and treatment:

Pulmonary function: moderate COPD with an FEV_1 of 1.56 L (51% of normal), total lung capacity of 7.66 L (116% of normal), maximal voluntary ventilation of 81 L/min (72% of normal), and a normal diffusing capacity and arterial oxygen saturation

Echocardiogram: normal left ventricular size and function with an LVEF of 50%; borderline concentric left ventricular hypertrophy; severe calcific aortic stenosis with an aortic valve area of 0.7 cm^2 and a mean gradient of 49 mmHg

Coronary angiogram: mild obstructive coronary artery disease with 40% stenosis in the distal left anterior descending and proximal circumflex coronary arteries. The patient was placed on captopril 12.5 mg tid and continued on Dyazide one tablet qd, aspirin 325 mg qd, and Maxair inhaler 2 puffs qid

Cardiopulmonary exercise testing: This was carried out to assess the clinical severity of the patient's valvular lesion. Treadmill exercise time was 4.3 minutes to a speed of 1.5 mph and a grade of 7.0% with a limiting symptom of dyspnea. Heart rate increase was from 92-144 beats/min; blood pressure increased from 156/70 to 178/66. The electrocardiogram revealed no significant arrhythmias and was interpreted as nondiagnostic for myocardial ischemia secondary to voltage criteria for left ventricular hypertrophy. Pulmonary responses to exercise were normal with a breathing reserve of 25 L/min and no arterial desaturation detected by oximetry. The $\dot{V}O_2$peak was 1.6 L/min, 17.9 ml/kg/min or 5.1 METs (87% of normal for age and gender). However, a plateau in the $\dot{V}O_2$ curve was seen at peak exercise (respiratory exchange ratio of 1.18) consistent with a cardiac output limitation to exercise.

Cardiac Rehabilitation Consultation
The patient was referred for a possible supervised exercise program. At present, the patient performs usual activities of daily living including walking stairs at home (tri-level house) and performing the shopping tasks for the family, but has no formal exercise program.

Risk Stratification for Exercise Training
Significant aortic stenosis with a plateau in oxygen uptake during symptom-limited exercise, implying an abnormal cardiac output limitation. Overall risk: moderate to high

Cardiac Rehabilitation Models
Model D or E

Exercise Prescription
An ECG-monitored program for two to three weeks will be started. If all goes well, the patient will then be moved to a nonmonitored program (phase III) or a combination of phase III and home exercise training with a total exercise frequency of 3-5 sessions per week. A target heart rate of 120-132 beats/min (60% to 70% of the heart rate reserve), and perceived exertion ratings of 12-14 (somewhat hard) will be prescribed to regulate exercise

intensity. Types of exercise may include walking, cycling, rowing, and so on, with special care to include some upper extremity exercise in each session. Exercise duration will begin at approximately 5-10 minutes per session and increase by up to 5 minutes each session to a goal duration of 30-45 minutes.

Case Study Number Eight

Congestive Heart Failure Secondary to Diastolic Dysfunction

The patient is a 73-year-old, married male, retired physicist (height 165 cm, weight 62.6 kg).

Past Medical History

Gout, hypertension, partial right knee menisectomy in 1981

Cardiovascular History

The patient experienced a subendocardial myocardial infarction in 1970. In 1976, he suffered an out-of-hospital cardiac arrest and his evaluation revealed significant two-vessel coronary artery disease and he underwent coronary bypass surgery (saphenous vein grafts to the right and circumflex coronaries).

In 1979, his previously normal resting electrocardiogram was found to have developed a left bundle branch block.

In 1984, he experienced his second myocardial infarction. At that time, his LVEF was 54%, his bypass grafts from his 1976 operation were patent, but significant obstructive disease was present in the left anterior descending and first diagonal branch vessels. He was managed with medical therapy, his recovery was uncomplicated, and he successfully completed a phase II cardiac rehabilitation program.

In 1994, he began to experience typical angina pectoris (substernal pain) with exertion and emotional stress. A heart catheterization demonstrated a LVEF of 52%, moderately elevated left ventricular end-diastolic pressure, significant obstructive disease in both saphenous vein grafts, moderate disease in the first diagonal branch, and a 95% proximal left anterior descending coronary artery lesion. Repeat coronary bypass surgery was performed with a left internal mammary artery graft to the left anterior descending, and saphenous vein grafts to the first diagonal, obtuse marginal branch of the circumflex, and the right coronary artery.

The patient entered the outpatient cardiac rehabilitation program and made an uneventful recovery. He participated in supervised exercise, walking and stationary cycling for up to 60 minutes three times per week without any cardiac symptoms. He attended educational classes, had a consultation with a cardiovascular dietitian, and participated in the patient/spouse support group with his wife. Coronary risk factors were assessed approximately six weeks after surgery and included the following:

Age

Gender

Hypertension (currently normal without any medication)

Positive family history (father and brother with coronary disease in their 50s)

Previous tobacco exposure (stopped cigarettes in 1970)

Hyperlipidemia (total cholesterol 226 mg/dl, high-density lipoprotein cholesterol 46 mg/dl, triglycerides 157 mg/dl, low-density lipoprotein cholesterol 149 mg/dl)

He responded well to the rehabilitation program. The dietitian felt that his dietary compliance was excellent, and he was started on a lipid-improving medication (lovastatin). He performed a symptom-limited treadmill test to a workload of 6.2 METs (measured $\dot{V}O_2$) and was moved into phase III cardiac rehabilitation approximately seven weeks after his bypass surgery. Medications at this time consisted of the following:

Lovastatin 20 mg qhs

Aspirin 81 mg qd

Allopurinol 100 mg bid

Blood lipids responded to the diet, exercise, and lovastatin with an LDL-C of 80 mg/dl, total-C 161 mg/dl, HDL-C 54 mg/dl and triglycerides 132 mg/dl approximately two months into the phase III program.

Approximately six months later the patient reported a gradual decline in his ability to perform his usual treadmill workout. He complained of dyspnea with only mild exertion and was seen by his cardiologist. His exam revealed bilateral rales and mild peripheral edema. An echocardiogram demonstrated normal left ventricular size with normal left ventricular systolic function (LVEF 50%) and evidence of an inferior wall myocardial infarction and paradoxical septal motion consistent with the patient's left bundle branch block and bypass surgery. However, pulmonary hypertension was found (right ventricular systolic pressure of 72 mmHg) and the diagnosis of diastolic dysfunction was made. The patient's exercise program was temporarily stopped and a calcium channel blocker (verapamil 40 mg tid) and diuretic (furosemide 20 mg qd) was started, but resulted in no improvement. Six weeks later an angiotensin-converting enzyme inhibitor (benazepril 5 mg qd) was begun and the calcium blocker discontinued.

Over the next two weeks the patient's symptoms improved and a cardiopulmonary exercise test was obtained. Treadmill time was 9.0 minutes with a peak speed of 3.0 mph and a grade of 17.5%. Heart rate increased from 80-150 beats/min and blood pressure from 164/90 to 194/60. The electrocardiogram was nondiagnostic for ischemia (LBBB) and there was no arrhythmia. Pulse oximetry revealed no significant arterial desaturation with exercise (96% to 93%). The $\dot{V}O_2$ curve plateaued at peak exercise, consistent with cardiac limitation, but the aerobic capacity was 19.9 ml/kg/min (5.7 METs) which was only slightly below his previous treadmill-measured exercise capacity. The patient returned to his exercise program.

Risk Stratification for Exercise Training
History of congestive heart failure secondary to diastolic dysfunction, pulmonary hypertension, plateau in $\dot{V}O_2$ consistent with cardiac output limitation (mild). Overall risk: moderate to high.

Cardiac Rehabilitation Model
Model D

Exercise Prescription
An initial ECG-monitored program (3-6 sessions) with subsequent phase III program with supplemental home exercise sessions, gradual return to usual exercise duration and intensity over a two- to four- week period, target heart rate 120-132 beats/min (55% to 70% of heart rate reserve).

Case Study Number Nine

Amyloid Heart Disease
This patient is a 53-year-old woman who is divorced, and whose occupation is a social worker (height 166 cm, weight 64.5 kg).

Past Medical History
Hysterectomy performed in 1978. Multiple myeloma diagnosed in 1989. Systemic amyloidosis diagnosed in 1991.

Cardiovascular History
Intermittent third degree AV block was discovered in 1992 with a subsequent permanent pacemaker implantation (DDDR, heart rate 60-120).

The patient's active lifestyle became compromised by progressive dyspnea on exertion and she was referred to a cardiologist by her oncologist for the question of cardiac disease. An echocardiogram showed a small left ventricular cavity with an ejection fraction of 73%. The ventricular walls were markedly thickened compatible with an infiltrative cardiomyopathy of amyloidosis.

Cardiac Rehabilitation Consultation

The patient was referred for a potential exercise training program. Medications consisted of the following:

Prednisone 60 mg qd

Dyazide one tablet bid

Alkeran 6 mg qd

Cholchicine 0.6 mg qd

Nifedipine XL 30 mg qd

Estrogen 0.625 mg qd

Folic acid 1 mg tid

A cardiopulmonary exercise test was performed for 3.6 minutes on the treadmill to a speed of 2.0 mph and a grade of 7.0%. Heart rate increased from 81-102 beats/min and blood pressure from 108/70 to 120/70. The electrocardiogram revealed a paced rhythm throughout the test. The $\dot{V}O_2$peak was 651 ml/min, 12.6 ml/kg/min, 3.5 METs (44.2% of age and gender predicted). Peak respiratory exchange ratio was 1.23. Pulmonary responses were within the normal limits.

Risk Stratification for Exercise Training

Extremely poor exercise capacity, amyloid cardiomyopathy. Overall risk: high

Cardiac Rehabilitation Model

Model B

Exercise Prescription

The patient will enter an ECG-monitored phase II program for a period of four to six weeks, with a phase III unmonitored program with supplemental home exercise sessions thereafter. Perceived exertion levels of 11-13 (fairly light to somewhat hard) will be used to regulate exercise intensity with an energy expenditure of 2 METs at the beginning of the program. A target heart rate will not be used due to the rate-responsive pacemaker (DDDR 60-120). Modes of activity will include cycle ergometry (including upper extremities) and treadmill walking. Because of the patient's poor exercise tolerance, initially an interval program (5-10 minutes exercise, 2-5 minutes rest, 2-4 repeats) will be used, although the goal will be to gradually increase continuous duration to 30-45 minutes per session. Repeat cardiopulmonary exercise testing will be performed in eight to 12 weeks to assess the patient's responses to the training program objectively.

Case Study Number Ten

Ischemic Cardiomyopathy, Malignant Ventricular Arrhythmia Treated With an ICD and Amiodarone

This male patient is 74 years old, is married, and retired from cheesemaking approximately ten years ago (height 182 cm, weight 73.7 kg).

Past Medical History

Hypertension, a generalized anxiety disorder with no specific treatment, mild COPD, FEV_1 2.34 L (73% of normal).

Cardiovascular History

The patient experienced a witnessed out-of-hospital cardiac arrest, was successfully resuscitated and transported to the emergency room. The diagnosis of an acute inferior wall myocardial infarction was made. Mild anoxic encephalopathy was present but resolved within five days. An echocardiogram demonstrated an LVEF of 35% with inferior wall hypokinesis and mild mitral valve regurgitation. Coronary angiography was performed with the findings of a right dominant circulation with an occluded mid right coronary artery and moderate obstructive disease in the left anterior descending. An electrophysiological study revealed inducible sustained, poorly tolerated polymorphic ventricular tachycardia.

An implantable cardioverter-defibrillator was placed transvenously (nonthoracotomy placement). Frequent episodes of ventricular tachycardia and ventricular fibrillation resulted in appropriate device discharges. Therefore, amiodarone was instituted. In four weeks of follow-up after starting the antiarrythmic drug, only one device discharge occurred.

A dipyridamole thallium perfusion scan was obtained that demonstrated a fixed inferior wall defect consistent with infarction and no evidence of ischemia.

Cardiac Rehabilitation Consultation

The patient was referred for an exercise program and secondary prevention efforts. Medications consisted of the following:

Amiodarone 400 mg qd

Metoprolol 25 mg bid

Losartan 75 mg qd

Aspirin 325 mg qd

Coronary risk factors were reviewed and are as follows:

Age

Gender

Previous tobacco exposure (stopped cigarettes 11 years previously, 26 pack-year exposure)

Hypertension (controlled medically)

Adverse blood lipid profile (total cholesterol 223 mg/dl, HDL-C 36 mg/dl, LDL-C 151 mg/dl, triglycerides 182 mg/dl)

Stress (anxious, difficulty sleeping since the cardiac event)

Sedentary lifestyle

The patient and spouse will be encouraged to see the dietitian for instruction and follow-up of a low-fat diet. Body weight and composition are reasonable at present (21% fat by skinfold measurements). Repeat blood lipids will be performed in eight weeks with an LDL-C goal of < 100 mg/dl. Educational classes dealing with coronary artery disease and the support group will be offered to the patient and spouse.

Due to the patient's obvious psychological distress, a referral to a psychiatrist will be made.

Risk Stratification for Exercise Training
Depressed left ventricular ejection fraction, inducible malignant ventricular arrhythmia treated with an implantable defibrillator, and an antiarrhythmic medication. Overall risk: high

Cardiac Rehabilitation Program Models
Model A (initially), when safety of exercise training is established the patient could move to Model B, D, or E

Exercise Prescription
A phase II ECG-monitored program will be implemented and continued for a period of four to eight weeks, with a frequency of three to four sessions per week, to assess the patient's responses to the training program. Care will be taken to keep the patient's exercise heart rate below the device's threshold rate for automatic cardioversion. An exercise test will not be performed and perceived exertion ratings of 12-14 (somewhat hard) will be used to regulate intensity. Modes of activity will be treadmill walking and cycle ergometry (no upper extremity exercise for four weeks per the cardiologist who implanted the ICD). Exercise duration will be gradually increased to 30-45 minutes per session (excluding warm-up and cool-down), as tolerated. After a period of weeks of incident-free exercise training in the supervised program, some supplemental home exercise sessions will be added to the program. A long-term phase III supervised, but unmonitored program will

be recommended. Repeat stress testing will be left to the discretion of the patient's cardiologist.

Case Study Number Eleven

Myocardial Ischemia Assessed by Exercise Radionuclide Angiography Without Chest Pain or Electrocardiographic Abnormalities

The patient is a 49-year-old, divorced man who works as a social worker for a government agency (height 175 cm, weight 98.6 kg).

Past Medical History
Type II diabetes mellitus diagnosed in 1987.

Cardiovascular History
An inferior wall myocardial infarction occurred in 1989. A cardiac catheterization performed at that time demonstrated an occluded mid RCA, a 40% proximal LAD stenosis, a 30% proximal circumflex lesion, and a left ventricular ejection fraction of 58%. The patient was treated medically and did well for several years.

In November of this year, the patient was hospitalized with rapid onset dyspnea at rest and was found to have suffered an acute lateral wall myocardial infarction. Emergent treatment included thrombolysis (tissue plasminogen activator) as well as a coronary angiogram that showed the previously occluded RCA, a 90% proximal circumflex lesion, and a 70% mid LAD stenosis. Balloon angioplasty and two stents were successfully applied to the circumflex lesion. The patient's subsequent four-day hospital stay was uneventful. Medical treatment included the following:

Metformin 500 mg bid

Aspirin 325 mg qd

Metoprolol 50 mg bid

Ticlopidine 250 mg bid (for two weeks)

Approximately two weeks after hospital dismissal, the patient returned to his cardiologist, who felt that the patient was angina- and dyspnea-free and doing well. An exercise radionuclide angiogram (MUGA) was performed to evaluate left ventricular function at rest and during each stage of an incremental supine cycling exercise test (see table 5.3). The following data were obtained:

Table 5.3   Myocardial Ischemia Assessed by Exercise Radionuclide Angiography

Exercise stage	Rest	300 kpm/min	600 kpm/min	900 kpm/min
Heart rate, beats/min	64	82	97	119
Blood pressure, mmHg	106/64	142/80	174/96	166/102
Rate-pressure product	6,784	11,644	16,878	19,754
LVEF, %	41	43	40	28

Symptoms: leg fatigue and moderate dyspnea, which were the reasons for test termination.

Electrocardiogram: less than 1 mm horizontal ST segment depression in leads V4-V5 at peak exercise, interpretation was negative for ischemia

Left ventricular function: at rest, hypokinesis of the inferior, inferolateral, and lateral walls was present with an LVEF of 41%. During the first two stages of exercise (300 and 600 kpm/min), global and regional left ventricular function was well-maintained. At peak exercise (900 kpm/min), additional severe hypokinesis of the anterior wall was noted with a decrease in LVEF to 28%, consistent with exercise-related myocardial ischemia involving the anterior wall.

The cardiologist felt that the LAD was not amenable to angioplasty and offered the patient a consultation with a cardiothoracic surgeon for consideration of coronary bypass surgery, but the patient declined. Lisinopril 5 mg qd was added to the patient's medical program.

Cardiac Rehabilitation Consultation
The patient was referred for a supervised exercise program and aggressive coronary risk reduction. Coronary risk factors included the following:

Gender

Type II diabetes mellitus

Previous tobacco use (stopped cigarettes in 1989, 22 pack-year exposure)

Mild hyperlipidemia, total cholesterol 206 mg/dl, HDL-C 31 mg/dl, LDL-C 132 mg/dl, triglycerides 216 mg/dl

Obesity, 98.6 kg (217 lbs), 28% body fat by skinfold assessment, waist-to-hip ratio 0.99 (central obesity)

Psychosocial stress with recent divorce and loss of custody of two teenage children

Sedentary lifestyle

The patient's primary physician had been closely following the diabetes and a recent glycosylated hemoglobin level was 8.2%, indicating fairly good glycemic control. The patient's metformin dose was not altered. However, the patient was at least 25 lbs overweight and will see the dietitian and attend the diet classes with follow-up as needed.

Blood lipids will be treated with diet, exercise, and weight control for three months and then the lipid profile will be measured again. Goals include an LDL-C < 100 mg/dl, HDL-C > 35 mg/dl, triglycerides < 200 mg/dl. Lipid-improving medication, such as simvastatin, may be required for achievement of these goals. Because of the patient's young age and relatively benign blood lipid profile, a plasma homocysteine level will be determined and treated with folic acid and vitamins B6 and B12 if the concentration is > 10 µmol/L.

A psychosocial assessment using the Symptom Checklist 90-R will be performed and the patient referred to a behavioral medicine specialist for stress-reduction training and eating behavior modification. Depending upon the result of the psychosocial evaluation, the patient may be referred to a psychiatrist.

The patient will be encouraged to attend all of the patient education classes dealing with coronary artery disease and risk factor modification as well as the support group. Follow-up consultations with the patient's case manager will occur several times over the next six months.

The patient has not been physically active for many years. In the summer, he performs yard work once per week. He has no physically demanding hobbies and plays no sports. He acknowledges that his primary physician had implored him to begin a walking program as part of the treatment for diabetes, but that he had never been able to comply for more than a few days.

Risk Stratification for Exercise Training

Electrocardiographically and symptomatically silent myocardial ischemia, moderately depressed left ventricular systolic function. Overall risk: moderate to high

Cardiac Rehabilitation Models

Model B, D, or E would be appropriate, depending upon the patient's response to changing his exercise habits and willingness to continue in a long-term supervised exercise program.

Exercise Prescription

The patient should initially start an ECG-monitored phase II program for two or more weeks, until his self-assessment skills are developed and his confidence in his ability to exercise is adequate. Three supervised sessions per week will be prescribed with two unsupervised sessions per week at the outset of the program. The usual diabetic precautions concerning exercise will be reviewed. After two or more weeks of supervised exercise with monitoring, the patient will be moved to unmonitored status and will be encouraged to exercise at least five days per week and given the opportunity to continue in a phase III program or have telephone contact periodically with program personnel.

The patient demonstrated a substantial amount of myocardial ischemia during the exercise radionuclide angiogram. The standard techniques of calculating a target heart rate below the ischemic threshold are not possible in this case due to the following factors: no ST segment changes on the ECG, no symptoms of angina pectoris (to serve as a guide for the onset of ischemia); the heart rate response to supine exercise on the radionuclide angiogram is different than the heart rate response would be to upright exercise such as walking or cycling (making the heart rate reserve technique for calculating the target heart rate unreliable). However, one may use the rate-pressure product (a sensitive indicator of myocardial oxygen requirement) at the work intensity just below the ischemic threshold as an upper limit guide for exercise intensity. At peak exercise with a rate-pressure product of 19,754, the LVEF dropped and new regional wall-motion abnormalities were observed, consistent with myocardial ischemia. At the exercise stage just below peak exercise the rate-pressure product was 16,878, and the LVEF and regional wall motion were not much different from resting conditions, consistent with a lack of substantial myocardial ischemia. Therefore, for exercise intensity prescription for this patient, perceived exertion ratings of 12-14 (somewhat hard) will be prescribed with an upper limit rate-pressure product of 16,878. During the initial monitored exercise sessions, the heart rate and systolic blood pressure responses will be assessed and a more specific target heart rate may be determined for the patient corresponding to a desirable level of perceived exertion and rate-pressure product.

The modes of exercise for the patient will include walking, cycle ergometry (including arm and leg exercise), and upper extremity isotonic strengthening with handheld weights (3-10 lbs). Duration of exercise will start at ten minutes per session plus warm-up and cool-down activities, and will increase 3-5 minutes per session until a goal of 45 minutes per session is achieved.

References

Agency for Health Care Policy and Research; National Heart, Lung, and Blood Institute. U.S. Department of Health and Human Services; Public Health Service. 1995. *Clinical Practice Guideline Number 17: Cardiac Rehabilitation* (AHCPR Publication No. 96-0672). Washington, DC: U.S. Government Printing Office.

American Association of Cardiovascular and Pulmonary Rehabilitation. 1995. *Guidelines for Cardiac Rehabilitation Programs.* 2nd ed. Champaign, IL: Human Kinetics.

American College of Cardiology. 1986. Position report on cardiac rehabilitation. *J Am Coll Cardiol* 7:451-453.

American College of Physicians. 1988. Position paper: Cardiac rehabilitation services. *Ann Intern Med* 109:671-673.

American College of Sports Medicine. 1995. *ACSM's Guidelines for Exercise Testing and Prescription.* 5th ed. Baltimore: Williams & Wilkins.

Borg GAV. 1973. Perceived exertion: A note on "history" and methods. *Med Sci Sports* 5:90-93.

Chicharro JL, Sanchez O, Bandres F, Guantes Y, Yges A, Lucia A, Legido JC. 1994. Platelet aggregability in relation to the anaerobic threshold. *Thromb Res* 75:251-257.

Fletcher GF, Balady G, Froelicher VF, Hartley LH, Haskell WL, Pollock ML. 1995. Exercise standards: A statement for health care professionals from the American Heart Association. *Circulation* 91:580-615.

Hanson P. 1994. Exercise testing and training in patients with chronic heart failure. *Med Sci Sports Exerc* 26:527-537.

Hatcher KK, Brubaker PH, Rejeski WJ, Bergey DB, Miller HS. 1995. The safety and efficacy of exercise prescription in silent ischemia patients. *Med Sci Sports Exerc* 27:S218.

Kelly TM. 1995. Exercise testing and training of patients with malignant ventricular arrhythmias. *Med Sci Sports Exerc* 28:53-61.

Keteyian SJ, Mellett PA, Fedel FJ, McGowan CM, Stein PO. 1995. Electrocardiographic monitoring during cardiac rehabilitation. *Chest* 107:1242-1246.

Lee AP, Ice R, Blessy R, Sanmarco ME. 1979. Long-term effects of physical training on coronary patients with impaired ventricular function. *Circulation* 60:1519-1526.

Maybaum S, Ilan M, Mogilevsky J, Tzivoni D. 1996. Improvement in ischemic parameters during repeated exercise testing: A possible model for myocardial preconditioning. *Am J Cardiol* 78:1087-1091.

Meyer K, Roskamm H. 1997. What is the best training method for improving aerobic capacity in chronic heart failure patients? *Heart Failure* Summer:83-91.

Osborn MJ. 1996. Mechanisms, incidence, and prevention of sudden cardiac death. In *Mayo Clinic Practice of Cardiology.* 3rd ed. Giuliani ER, Gersh BJ, McGoon MD, Hayes DL, Schaff HV (eds). St. Louis: Mosby, pp. 862-894.

Pashkow FJ, Dafoe WA (eds). 1993. *Clinical Cardiac Rehabilitation: A Cardiologist's Guide.* Baltimore: Williams & Wilkins.

Pollock ML, Welsch MA, Graves JE. 1995. Exercise prescription for cardiac rehabilitation. In *Heart Disease and Rehabilitation*. 3rd ed. Pollock ML, Schmidt DH (eds). Champaign, IL: Human Kinetics, pp. 243-276.

Squires RW. 1985. Moderate altitude exposure and the cardiac patient. *J Cardiopulm Rehabil* 5:421-426.

Squires RW, Lavie CJ, Brandt TR, Gau GT, Bailey KR. 1987. Cardiac rehabilitation in patients with severe ischemic left ventricular dysfunction. *Mayo Clin Proc* 62:997-1002.

Squires RW, Miller TD, Harn T, Michaels TA, Palma TA. 1991a. Transtelephonic electrocardiographic monitoring of cardiac rehabilitation exercise sessions in coronary artery disease. *Am J Cardiol* 67:962-964.

Squires RW, Muri AJ, Anderson LJ, Allison TG, Miller TD, Gau GT. 1991b. Weight training during phase II (early outpatient) cardiac rehabilitation: Heart rate and blood pressure responses. *J Cardiopulm Rehabil* 11:360-364.

Stewart RAH, Simmonds MB, Williams MJA. 1995. Time course of "warm up" in stable angina. *Am J Cardiol* 76:70-73.

Sullivan MJ. 1994. New trends in cardiac rehabilitation in patients with chronic heart failure. *Prog Cardiovasc Nursing* 9:13-21.

White RD. 1996. Out-of-hospital intervention in sudden cardiac death. In *Mayo Clinic Practice of Cardiology*. 3rd ed. Giuliani ER, Gersh BJ, McGoon MD, Hayes DL, Schaff HV (eds). St. Louis: Mosby, pp. 895-907.

Index

REHABILITATION RESOURCES FOR CARDIOPULMONARY PROFESSIONALS

1996 • Cloth • 424 pp
Item BSOT0766
ISBN 0-87322-766-2
$36.00 ($53.95 Canadian)

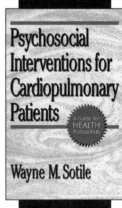

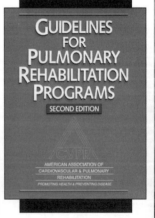

1998 • Paper • 152 pp
Item BFAR0536
ISBN 0-87322-536-8
ISSN 1071-7889
$24.00 ($35.95 Canadian)

1998 • Paper • 232 pp
Item BAAC0863
ISBN 0-88011-863-6
$35.00 ($52.50 Canadian)

To place your order, U.S. customers call TOLL FREE 1-800-747-4457. Customers outside the U.S. place your order using the appropriate telephone number/address shown in the front of this book.

HUMAN KINETICS

The Information Leader in Physical Activity
http://www.humankinetics.com/

2335